BIOTONICS

are no-sweat, no-time exercises
that can make you trimmer, stronger
and more energetic than you've ever
been in your entire adult life.

BIOTONICS

can be done anytime, anywhere: sitting
at your desk, waiting in your car for
the light to change, while you read,
when you shower or as you watch TV.

- These powerful, six-second muscle contractions performed once a day can build maximum stamina in just twelve weeks.

- These motion exercises can keep your joints supple and youthful so that you can use them without pain or injury.

- Combined with Dr. Wiederanders' tested, high-protein diet, BIOTONICS can help you slim down.

DETAILED LINE DRAWINGS ILLUSTRATE EACH EXERCISE!

CHARTS ENABLE YOU TO TAILOR A FULL EXERCISE PROGRAM TO FIT YOUR NEEDS

BIOTONICS

BIOTONICS

Stamina Through Six-Second
Exercises That Really Work

REX E. WIEDERANDERS, M.D.
with Edmond G. Addeo

WARNER BOOKS

A Warner Communications Company

To the Carole in my heart

WARNER BOOKS EDITION

Library of Congress Catalog Card Number 77-8208

ISBN 0-446-82838-6

This Warner Books Edition is published by
arrangement with Harper & Row, Inc.

Cover design by New Studio

Warner Books, Inc., 75 Rockefeller Plaza, New York, N.Y. 10019

Ⓦ A Warner Communications Company

Printed in Canada

Not associated with Warner Press, Inc. of Anderson, Indiana

First Printing: November, 1978

10 9 8 7 6 5 4 3 2 1

Acknowledgments

The fact that everybody eats and exercises seems to make everybody an expert in the fields of nutrition and exercise. Fortunately for our good health and sanity, there are a few *real* experts.

For particular commendation I would like to single out my long-term friend, Dr. Gary Evans, of the Human Nutrition Laboratories, Grand Forks, North Dakota. Gary has distinguished himself as the outstanding American authority on trace minerals. He knows more about what goes into the human mouth and what happens to it than anyone I know. His advice and comments on the manuscript have been most valuable.

Also, I would like to mention Steve Hughes, physical therapist from Mercy Hospital, Williston, North Dakota. Steve supplied from his own excellent library a number of the references I have found helpful. He was also kind enough to share with me many of the personal experiences he has had in his work as physical therapist.

R.E.W.

CONTENTS

PART ONE

How the Biotonic Strength and Stamina Program Works

CHAPTER 1

Your Muscles:
The Fountains of Youth

Congratulations. You've already taken the first step to better physical conditioning: you have committed yourself. You wouldn't be reading this book if you didn't think you needed a new avenue for physical improvement. You *know* you could be in better shape, have more stamina, feel better more often. You have admitted to needing more vigor, more vitality, more physical self-confidence when beginning an activity, better *performance* from the muscles and bones which make up the incredible machine that is your body. And because of this, I'm not going to ask if you think you're "inactive" when I mean "lazy"; I'm not going to query you on being "soft" when I mean "fat." It's your body, your life. You have to live within your own body, no one else's. All other things being equal, you alone control whether when you retire you'll be an active, strong, agile person who enjoys physical recreation and feeling good *all the time,* or whether you'll be stiff and decrepit, unable to swing a golf club or walk farther than fifty yards at a time.

You've made the first step by opening the cover of this book. What I can now promise you is that if you undertake a regular, daily program of the exercises outlined in later chapters, you will be a better physical specimen *for a greater number of years* than you would have otherwise thought possible.

Think of this. Animals are healthier, more active and more supple for a far greater percentage of their lifetime than human beings. A cat, for example, is muscularly supple and lithe for almost ⅞ of its life. A human being, on the other hand, is only considered in "prime condition" for about half his life.

Why is that? The answer is simple, if you've spent time watching a cat. See how often he stretches. See him wake from a nap and stretch every muscle and work every joint in his body. Stretching his paws and hind legs, arching his back and curving the spine . . . a lithe, healthy creature able to perform amazing feats of physical activity for ⅞ of his life. And you? How often have you taken just a minute to touch your toes a few times? (Can't? Then go as far as you *can!*) How often do you flex your biceps, your forearms, wriggle your wrists and ankles, bend over backward to compress those vertebrae, do a deep knee bend or two? How long does it take?

How long will ⅞ of *your* life be? And what will be its quality? Will you be young, in possession of good blood vessels and snug joints, trim and svelte, glowing with life, or will you be a candidate for the old age home before your life has really gotten underway? The old age home? Visit one. See what cheer fills its halls. Notice how many of those souls are of sound mind but crippled body, sitting out the game of life when they should still be playing.

Will ⅘ of your life be spent sheathed in fat, moving like a ponderous yacht? Will you be like so many patients we surgeons see nowadays? The picture returns like a nightmare. There lies the massive body, clothed in fat so deep you cannot find the person inside. This body sticks up so far above the table that platforms have to be ordered for even the tall surgeons to stand on. And it's necessary to cut and cut and the fat goes on forever.

I remember one patient so well. He had sufficient muscle to hold together the barrel of fat that he carried, but the moment we got inside we could scarcely find his organs. Each one was enveloped by fat, like thick insulation, great, knobby lumps of it. And we tugged and strained and the interns pulled and the surgeon cursed and swore and the nurses grunted to get the necessary exposure. Certainly he was on the table at least twice as long as he needed to be. All that extra time under anaesthetic and just because he was fat.

His danger during surgery was at least twice that of a thin patient, and his complication risk ten times that of the slender man. Of course, he broke open his wound after surgery and ended up with ugly wire sutures holding him together. His wound was slow to heal and he finally ended up with a hernia which he is too fat to have repaired. He is like a barrelful of lard and this lard is incompressible. Every time he coughs or sneezes he exerts tension all over his belly. There is no room for anything but that fat. One wonders how he can eat at all, but apparently nature has ordained that even the morbidly obese can still eat.

Morbidly obese. The phrase refers to those so fat they can do little but waddle around and vegetate. They sit a lot and gather more fat and lose the one hope they have: their muscle strength.

This book represents a new approach to building and maintaining your muscular strength, your stamina and endurance, your overall body tone, and suggests a sensible diet for reaching and maintaining your ideal weight. The average American is currently preoccupied with looking good, with getting into shape, with exercise—which is fine. The TV addict, the overeater, the lazy slug, the softie, they all need *something* and it's slightly heartening to see that a few more Americans than before are turning to some sort of physical fitness program to halt the steady decline of their physical and mental well-being. Weight-watching combined with jogging, tennis, swimming and a host of other programs is steadily gaining in popularity, and indeed the fear of heart attack, emphysema, high blood pressure and other debilitating diseases has encouraged the American male and female to take up almost every activity from belly dancing to marathon running.

But what about stamina? Does it do a person any good to simply "look good"? Is anything happening in our muscular systems that the fad diets, weekend sports and trendy new meditative schemes are ignoring? To answer that we have to look at how we've been conditioned—or, more accurately, de-conditioned—by our life styles.

To say America is becoming a nation of lazy slobs would be cruel and unkind—and a cliché. But, like all clichés, there is a lot of truth in it. We are now fitted with trail bikes, golf carts, motorcycles, cars, buses, trains, planes and, Lord help us, even snowmobiles! For most of our adult lives we have been letting gasoline or electricity do most of our work. We don't walk to whatever recreation we do have, we don't walk to work. We don't walk to our personal affairs, we don't walk to the library, we don't walk to visit friends. Our entire lives are spent sitting down and being propelled from place to place.

The price of progress. Of course, a man in Brooklyn can't be expected to walk to his office in Manhattan. A man in Chicago can't be expected to jog his way to Joliet. And if we eliminated the freeways in Los Angeles we wouldn't necessarily have healthier people, we'd have a ghost town!

Yes, there is justification for this apparent victimization by "progress." We have no time. The successful business person today is the hyper-hyped man or woman "on the go," the airplane commuter, the chauffeured executive, the young tyro in his sports car. To get ahead, we must dictate into exotic electronic equipment, shunning even our writing muscles. (I have a writer friend who dictates his articles and books onto tapes, or else types two-fingeredly on an electric typewriter and whose handwriting has consequently degenerated into a hieroglyphic scrawl.) We take elevators, escalators and even "moving sidewalks" in our airports. We carry neither our luggage nor our groceries. A major international business machine corporation even advertises, "Machines should work; people should think." A truly obscene slogan!

In short, we do everything possible to save time, because there doesn't seem to be enough time in

17

the day (even to think?). And in the process we are letting our muscles soften into pasty flab.

To compound this sedentary collapse we eat a weird combination of foods made largely of fat and carbohydrates, of *refined* sugar and starch, fast foods that are available in an instant to accommodate our instant lives. These things are artificial and largely stripped of any real nutritional value, and we've made them our daily fare. We eat them semiprone in front of that ubiquitous mind drag, the TV set. So from machine to machine we go, getting softer and softer, sicker and sicker, until we fabricate our own personal disaster in the form of "shaping up."

This is our rebellion. "I'm going to get in shape and start exercising, not like those other guys." So we get out and jog and run and throw our bowling balls and swing our drivers and softball bats and rackets and we work up "a good sweat." Boy, do we feel good! The next day we hurt like hell, our heads are groggy and our bodies feel like dishrags. Maybe we've pulled a muscle or twisted a joint or sprained an ankle. But we worked up that "good sweat." *We got some exercise!*

(Some of us, a pitiful few, *have* developed a good exercise regimen and stick to it intelligently. This discussion is not aimed at them, although they, too, can benefit from the strength and stamina exercises outlined in this book. There is no upper limit to what can be gained.)

So, for the following week, off we go, swilling our two martinis before lunch and three before dinner, slouching on padded and contoured couches, letting our muscles fall into complete sloth in the armchair of success—until the next weekend. Then we get all fired up again and work up that "good sweat."

What is this doing to our bodies? It is nearly wrecking them. We are asking a machine used to doing the barest minimum of work with a minimum of maintenance to throw its full force into exercises and exertions that would strain a professional athlete. A heart that pumps five liters per minute in the normal course of daily life is suddenly asked to pump twice that amount, that is, to do twice the work in the same amount of time. An incredible strain. It's exactly like picking up one hundred pounds in a single jerk, having been used to picking up only fifty.

Your heart, starved for protein, lacking in vitamins, full of plastic substances and false foods, is suddenly asked to do twice its accustomed work. Itself a pale bag of flapping muscles, the heart is forced to its utmost as we Walter Mittys try in vain to transform ourselves into Roscoe Tanner, Jack Nicklaus, Dorothy Hammil, Nadia Comanici and Frank Shorter all rolled into one. And, of course, we work up that "good sweat."

"Good sweat?" Good grief! Is it any wonder our weekend athletes drop dead under the broiling afternoon sun? Is it any wonder that sprained ankles, sunstroke, broken limbs, twisted joints, pulled tendons, strokes, coronaries, dislocated shoulders and charley horses are plaguing the nation's streets, parks, resorts and playing fields? Ah, but when they hit the ground, those flabby, soft, veiny-legged weekend warriors, they are beautifully bathed from sunburned face to stubby toe in that "good sweat."

Of course, the heart is the glamor-boy of the

body. It gets the headlines—along with the brain—while the other muscles make page twenty-six. But the heart is only a muscle, like the rest. And the rest—*all* the muscles!—are also suddenly flushed with hot new blood as the arteries open and the veins respond under punishing physical activity. Muscles that complain about mowing the lawn or shoveling snow and rarely move more than a centimeter are now suddenly pushed through great extremes of exertive activity. Even worse, joints feebly protected by pale, weak muscles are banged around like loose, clanging gears in a box without oil.

It's a well-recognized, widely-preached doctrine: *get in shape before you exert yourself!* Ask any coach, any physical therapist. This is what "getting in shape" is all about, strengthening your muscles to pull the joints tightly into their sockets in order to *protect* as well as to move your body.

A joint is a mechanical bearing, no more, no less. Any bearing set tightly with exact tolerances and good lubrication will last a long time. Conversely, any loose and clattering bearing must wear out quickly. The weekend athlete takes these loose and clattering joints to the handball court and beats the lining out of them. And they ache the next day, and they will ache after each such punishment. This ache is trying to tell you something, that the joint surface is getting rough and putting small bits of itself afloat in the joint fluid. It is dying. It could be destroyed.

The joints are not the only system damaged by unprepared exertion. When the heart suddenly demands *all* the blood, it sends out adrenalin and nonadrenalin to marshal its reserves. The arteries to the stomach, intestines and liver then constrict or even close completely and these organs must limp along on a miniscule amount of nutrients. The poor spleen squeezes down like a pale sponge to give up as much blood as it can. This causes that familiar pain in the left side just under the ribs. Is it any wonder we leave the playing field nauseated, bilious, headachey and miserable?

Many of us take what we think is a more reasonable view. We trudge off to the links or courts with our friends and compete on a regular basis. We have compact, enduring bodies, our joints are tight and stable, muscles firm, ready to drive us. Even our guts and lungs are seasoned. We are fit: but we have lonely, frustrated mates and rebellious kids who wonder in their numb way why they hardly ever see their father or mother.

Between these two extremes comes the great compromise. We cut down on our TV time and take the kids skating or to play tennis, whatever. This lasts a day. Or we give up our lunch hour and plunge into a handball game and a sauna, go back to work feeling like a massaged sponge and fall asleep. None of these expedients can last. There just is not a certain time regularly set aside each day for exercise. "If only I had an extra hour every day," we moan as we rush through life and promise ourselves a better tomorrow. We promise ourselves we'll start an exercise routine, we'll "get in shape and *stay* there," we'll whip our bodies into condition . . . when we get time.

Well, here's the *good* news. There *is* time. You will find with this exercise program that there are no uniforms to buy, no sweat suits to wear, no pills to pop, no weights to lift, no apparatus or equipment to maintain . . . nothing is required but your own body. And you can do almost any exercise in this book anywhere, at any time. Got a minute between phone calls? Waiting for someone to drop by? Between that last cup of coffee and the housecleaning? Waiting for a bus? A train? Do a few of the less visible exercises. Taking a shower? Don't wash your tummy until it's contracted—and keep it there! Putting on your shoes? Your tie? Waiting for the car to warm up? Waiting for a tennis court? Picking the kids up from school? Sitting down to write a letter? Watching TV? Walking up—or down—the stairs? Alone in an elevator? Waiting in a supermarket line? The laundromat? The library? Getting gas? Hiking? Biking?

There. Count up all the time you really do have, even when you *seem* to be doing something. You'll find that my exercise theory will get you in shape in only those seconds and minutes each day, and keep you there. In the instances I mentioned above, you could have exercised—*made stronger*—almost every muscle in your body and almost every joint!

It seems that once we really set our minds to it, the very disease of our society itself, the sitting and standing around, doing nothing, can actually be used for our salvation. Because these exercises are designed to be of the "no-time, no-sweat" variety, we need no longer sit and vegetate at the whim of some steel monster. Waiting for the washing machine to stop? Why not take a minute to strengthen your arm muscles? Going out to pick up the mail? Why not strengthen those shoulder joints and guard against bursitis? Stopped in traffic on the way to or from work? Why not get those leg muscles in shape for this weekend's tennis match? Waiting at the checkout stand? You could firm up that fanny without a soul knowing about it!

22

With far less time and effort than you would believe possible, too. Look at the graph on page 25 that we have adapted from Dr. Erich A. Mueller's article, "Influence of Training and of Inactivity on Muscle Strength." *It shows clearly that only one maximal contraction lasting six seconds a day will allow you to reach one hundred percent of your maximal strength in only five weeks,* if you are originally at fifty percent of your maximum strength. Less intense effort of sixty-five percent of the maximal effort achieves the same goal in nine weeks. On the other hand, making several maximal contractions totalling thirty seconds a day cuts only one week off the overall time required to reach the goal. This shows that only six seconds a day is required to bring a muscle to maximal strength in close to minimal time—five weeks. *And if you continue the exercise for twelve weeks you can maintain that strength by exercising only once a week thereafter.* This is why I recommend a twelve-week exercise program in this book. And I will show you a series of exercises which you can do anywhere and which require almost no time—and absolutely no money.

After all, the average man and woman can't *afford* to belong to the Golden Doors or Vic Tanny club. They can't afford a tennis or swim club membership. They can't play games every day. The golf courses are crowded on weekends. Jogging is, really, a lot of trouble. So they are still eating too much and getting soft . . . and wishing they had time to get in shape.

Count the spare moments in your day, as I've tried to enumerate them above, and you'll come up with at least an extra hour. A golden gift, to use in sporadic segments—thirty seconds here, two minutes there—to get your heart and lungs stronger, your muscles firmer and more supple, and your joints tight, your mind alert, your spine resilient and flexible. Whatever kind of person you are according to the chart in Chapter Two, you can use these extra moments to tone your body, to build to new heights of stamina and physical performance, to strengthen your muscles and prolong your active physical life. My exercises can be done almost anywhere, as I said, and require no straining or sweating; many of them can be done inconspicuously in public. Breath control, deep breathing exercises and lung expansion can be done any time you feel like it.

I call these exercises "biotonics." "Bio" is a prefix, from the Greek *bios*, meaning "life"; "tonic" means that which invigorates or strengthens, restoring the health or tone of the body. Hence, "biotonics," a new kind of exercise that is designed to strengthen and add new stamina to almost any person's body with surprisingly little time commitment.

The variety, frequency, type and amount of these exercises you do will depend entirely on your daily routine and upon how determined you are to regain the perfect proportions and stamina of your youth.

Every skill from tiddlywinks to tennis, from backgammon to baseball, from dominoes to the decathlon, is preceded by the dull words, "Now remember, you can only learn by daily practice. A little each day, but it must be *every* day. Practice makes perfect." For those of you who are thoroughly familiar with this, omit the rest of this paragraph. But for those of you needing exhortation, remember, daily repetitions, every day, 365 days

Figure 1

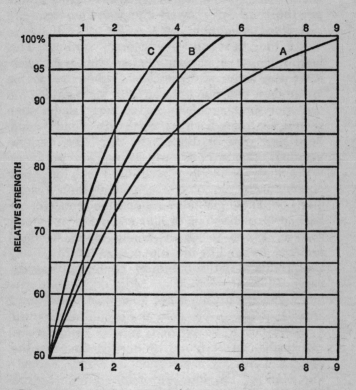

This shows the remarkable strength to be expected from only a short, maximal daily exertion. (A) sub-maximal, or sixty-five percent exertion daily; (B) one maximal daily contraction of only six seconds; (C) multiple daily maximal contraction totaling thirty seconds in duration.

a year, is the only way. Nothing but sore muscles and aching joints can result from only a few intense workouts once in a while. Patience and persistence are the babies that get you through and put the third "p"—power—into your muscles.

A Word of Caution.

It is time to sound a few general warnings. The first is to get a checkup before you start even these relatively easy exercises. Although doctors are human and our tests are still very crude, we can spot some problems in the early stages that should be treated with special care. Gout would head most lists of diseases to check for, as it is peculiarly sneaky in its early stages. Gout produces uric acid, an insoluble crystal that precipitates out of solution in the joints like meteors from a summer sky. These crystals lie along the tender cartilage surfaces like bits of flint and grind away the surface. When the body finally reacts to their presence by sending in white cells to destroy them, the products of the battle set up the violent inflammations of acute gout. Most doctors see patients with already neglected gout, with moth-eaten, arthritic joints, severe pain and disability. Gout, if its effects are to be avoided, must be found early.

Arthritis can be found by blood tests or in the blood and directly in the joints by X-rays. At least the joints of the four extremities and the neck should be put through their range of motion and checked for the grating, popping sound called crepitus. If this crepitus is present you know there is roughness in the joint. The usual cause of crepitus is some type of arthritis. Therefore, arthritis blood tests should be run and any joints under question X-rayed.

The heart should be carefully tested. Biotonic

26

exertions are short but intense, particularly the exertions of the chest and belly exercises. These exercises retard the blood return to the heart and can temporarily rob the heart and lungs of blood. The heart must be sound for this exertion. Recent improvements in testing allow a doctor to actually check the heart while the patient is exercising and much heart weakness can be found in this way that would otherwise be missed. Have a stress test run along with the enzyme studies that relate to heart function.

Another area of concern to the exerciser and dieter is the level of blood sugar. This should be spot-checked and a glucose tolerance test done if any questions arise. The high protein, natural foods recommended here are generally well tolerated by patients with both high blood sugar (diabetes) and "sugar shock," our term for hypoglycemia. Along with the blood sugar tests, modern laboratories offer a battery of other blood tests, checking calcium and cholesterol levels, among other things. Such a battery of tests is a good screening maneuver.

The lungs should be well tested. Vital capacity, or the amount of air that can be inhaled after a forced expiration, should be measured. Also the maximal breathing capacity should be determined. This is the total amount of air that can be breathed in and out in a given time. It is important that your lungs be functioning well for the breathing exercises. Consult your doctor before you start these.

The general status of the blood vessels should be noted. Do you have a good pulse in all extremities? Pulse is the indicator of blood flow in your arteries and you have to have a lot of blood for any kind of exercise, static thrust being no exception. How are your veins? Any varicose veins that might harbor a blood clot? A blood clot, which may also hide in the deep veins of the leg, can break off during exertion and travel to the lungs where it would cause sharp pains and sudden shortness of breath. This could be deadly but, if a clot is found ahead of time, there are medicines that can help dissolve it and lessen the danger. Exercise, of course, tends to prevent blood clot formation and this is now being encouraged for air travel, especially long distance flights during which the legs are subjected to long periods of immobility.

Another specific disease a doctor would be able to spot is epilepsy. This can be triggered by alterations in the blood components.

Other disabilities aggravated by exercise are hiatus hernia, a hidden weakness in the chest, and the more common groin hernia, but these would be picked up by a good physical. So, get a checkup first and be sure you have obtained your doctor's approval of your engaging in biotonic exercises before you start.

In the presentation of the exercises various safety facts are discussed when pertinent, but you must remember that all muscle strain, all forced breathing and even concentration change the patterns of blood flow to the brain. All exertion changes the amount of oxygen and sugar available to that delicate gelatin. Your brain cannot function even a minute without a supply of fresh oxygen. Therefore, *watch yourself*. Do not hold your breath or strain your muscles too long. The moment you feel the very first sign of dizziness or the beginning of that floating sensation that comes as a warning of lowered blood flow, stop the exercise and rest until you again feel normal.

One thing most of our exercises will not do per se is take off weight. One can walk briskly for nineteen minutes on the energy of one apple, jog fourteen minutes to burn up one martini. All the energy required for our exercises is probably found in one peanut. So do not be gulled. Do not kid yourself into thinking you can pile on extra food because you did your biotonic exercises. Not at all.

But these exercises can and will provide ideal conditioning exercise in preparation for more exuberant running and jumping sports and, by themselves, they will keep the joints supple and the muscles strong. Just being able to cut the lawn and weed the garden without being sore for a week is worth the price of admission.

And, again, these are exercises everyone can do and benefit from. Ladies and gentlemen are both invited. Active workers, athletes and sedentary workers at their desks and tables. White and blue collars, old and young. There are no specific body types, no medical classifications. Coronary Type A and Type B are invited and equally eligible under the rules described.

Now, let us get to the vexing question of smoking, although it would be very pleasant to avoid it completely. Too much money has already been poured into this fury. But we have to discuss it, as it affects the breathing exercises. In fact, it affects them so much that we do not recommend these exercises to smokers.

Smoking has an interesting effect on the lungs. It does not interfere with the actual volume of air the lungs can hold. This measurement, called the vital capacity, is normal in the smoker. But smoking does affect the *function* of the lungs. It affects the amount of air that can be moved through the lungs in a given time.

Apparently, smoking narrows the little tubes that carry air to the air sacs, the bronchioles. Narrow tubes mean more work and more time to move a given volume of air in and out of the lungs. The smoker can fill his lungs as deeply as the next guy but he can't do it as fast. He breaks down when he has to do this repeatedly against time. So repetitive breathing, forced breathing and controlled breathing are more difficult for the smoker and are more likely to cause temporary blackouts.

Well, here we go. I promise you you'll be a better physical person and you'll feel better *more often*, by the time you finish this book.

CHAPTER 2

Examination of Conscience: Designing Your Physical Goals

Just as no one can benefit from psychoanalysis unless he becomes perfectly honest with himself—and wants to benefit from it—no one can improve his physical condition unless he also makes a personal commitment to be perfectly candid about his *current* shape. You must first examine your conscience completely: *are* you lazy? Would you rather take the car to the store two blocks away, or would you enjoy walking? Have you started jogging and let it drop after a while because you'd rather stay snuggled in that warm bed in the morning, or have a glass of wine after work instead? Have you been *wanting* to get into shape, to start exercising, to take up yoga, to quit smoking, to give up bread or beer, to go on hikes with the family more often?

The answers to these and dozens of questions like them must be answered almost before you turn the page. You get out of exercise exactly what you put into it. You must decide now precisely where you are physically—being perfectly honest with yourself!—and where you want to be two, four, eight and twelve weeks from now. And because I am promising you that in twelve weeks you'll be a totally different physical being than you are now, I cannot overemphasize this point of determining exactly what shape you are in, your mental attitude and the *realistic* goals for which you should strive in the coming weeks. A man who wishes to get from point A to point C, but who knows full well he will falter and tend to stop at point B, must take that tendency into consideration when he is planning the trip. Consequently, if you've tried exercise programs before (as most of us have), but never really completed them, think about *why* you didn't. The RCAF exercises? Did you get all the way through and stay at your peak level? Any of the many diet fads? Did you lose the weight you wanted to lose and *keep* it off? That quit-smoking technique you tried? Are you still smoking?

Enough. My purpose isn't to lecture you into submission. You alone, as with the alcoholic who can't quit until he admits he needs outside help, must decide not only what you want out of this program, but also how badly you want it. In effect, you are deciding whether you want to be sluggish, overweight, soft and a pooper-outer, or whether you want to be youthful, vital, stronger, more dynamic and feel better *all the time*.

What can one reasonably expect to accomplish in this program? How does the program work?

The reasonable answer to the first question is as much as your inherent strength will allow. Therefore, when making the examination of conscience you have to consider your own physical stature and makeup. If you are a small-boned, slight person, you will not become a Primo Carnera. If you are a large, muscular sort, you are already strong and can add enormously to your strength. An active, long-distance runner can do himself only a comparatively slight good but a sedentary pencil pusher can virtually change his physical self overnight.

The answer to the second question is more complex and challenges our knowledge of muscle function. We know exercise is important for muscles but we also know they can exist without it. One could lie upon one's bed until he died of bed sores, until his muscles were but flaccid strings, but the muscles would still *be* there. Blood would flow to them, they would burn sugar; if properly exercised, they would even regain their former power. The muscles would not vanish. Even a minimum of activity keeps some function in the muscle.

But we also know that *effective* muscle function demands much more than minimal activity. The muscle must do more than just pull the joint around. It has to have *reserve* power. Power to snap that joint, cartilage to cartilage, and keep those surfaces snug as a fine watch. Power to glide those bones smoothly through their full range of motion. These are its basic tasks and it has to meet these easily and constantly. The muscle always has to be in a tense state to maintain that joint tension. If you are suddenly called upon to move, lift, jump, you have no time to tense your muscles and get ready. You want your muscles strong and tense *all* the time.

And you want plenty of reserve power. Power

to respond to any emergency, to do any out-of-the-ordinary task that may be asked of you—like moving furniture or carrying a heavy load. Particularly you want power and stamina for weekend recreation activities: golfing, tennis, skiing, surfing. Why should you have to end up on Sunday night with a mass of groaning joints and screaming muscles? This really is unnecessary. Power can be kept in the muscles at all times to do all tasks and meet all emergencies.

Should you be a weekend athlete? Should you run your heart out, work your legs numb and flail your arms and shoulders and neck about like wild toys? *Yes!* You bet you should. It is a medical axiom that sudden, *unaccustomed* strains on the heart can produce heart attacks and irregularities of the heart's rhythm that can lead to sudden death. In fact, a hot Sunday afternoon softball game killed one of my neighbors and left five nice people fatherless. At autopsy he was found to have poor coronary arteries, but he had actually electrocuted himself with his own heart electricity. An area of his heart muscle did not get enough blood for the strain he was putting on it; it started sending out electrical distress signals that overcame the usual, coordinated electrical system of his heart. These violent distress signals sent his heart into such a spasm—fibrillation as it's known medically—that it could not pump blood. A more gradual approach to physical activity—*especially on a hot day* —would probably have prevented it. But strenuous activity on the weekends is beneficial when sensibly pursued and prefaced by *some kind of physical conditioning*. This book aims to give you that conditioning easily and effectively.

You should have power in your muscles but, unlike your automobile, you cannot store power. You cannot have it unless you work for it steadily. The muscles will develop power in direct proportion to the demands made on them; the greater the demand, the greater the power. I have taken advantage of this fact by putting together a system of exercises that will continually increase your power, up to the full capacity of your muscle potential, and improve your stamina—because you are constantly working against yourself. The stronger you become the more strongly you oppose yourself and the stronger yet you can become.

Should you have this added strength? Do you need it? Absolutely. If you demand reserve power in your automobile and stereo, you certainly should demand it in yourself.

The point that a lot of us old die-hards find so totally unbelievable is that muscle power can be increased rapidly, steadily and to the fullest potential of the muscle without physical exhaustion, rivers of sweat, stinking locker rooms, chafing sweat suits or skin-ripping mats. In short, without noticeable *exertion*. Our German colleague Erich A. Mueller, M.D., a professor of physiology at the University of Muenster, Westfalen, and a member of the Max Planck Institute of Arbeitsphysiologie at Dortmund, has provided the medical community with a whole new outlook on muscle conditioning. He and his coworkers have debunked a vast number of misconceptions about muscle training and have laid down clear principles for our guidance. His methods give us reserve power so quickly and with such a small time investment that it seems unreal. But it works because a *static thrust* contraction is so much more powerful than anything that can be experienced in ordinary exercise. The concepts of Hellebrandt—exercising to exhaustion, making the muscles swell and ache and hurt, actually physically harming them—have been shown to produce stamina but are not necessary to build muscle strength. Strength is built by a powerful muscle contraction over a short period of time. Essentially the facts of Mueller's method are as follows:

1. All muscles strengthen in response to tension and can gain strength up to twelve percent per week.

2. This tension need be applied for only *six seconds a day* for five to nine weeks to achieve maximal strength of the muscle.

3. But, the tension must be greater than sixty percent of the muscle's total strength.

4. If exercise is stopped before twelve weeks the muscle weakens at about seven percent per day.

5. If exercise is stopped after twelve weeks and *only one exercise period a week* done thereafter, the muscle can be maintained at maximal strength.

6. Stamina is a direct function of strength. One can exert fifteen percent of his total strength indefinately, fifty percent of total strength for only one minute and *total* muscle strength for six seconds or less. For instance, if a subject can lift 100 lbs., then he can hold up 15 lbs. indefinitely, 50 lbs. for a minute and 100 lbs. for six seconds. If he doubles his strength, he can hold up 30 lbs. indefinitely, 100 lbs. for a full minute and 200 lbs. for six seconds. So his stamina has also doubled. Strength and stamina march hand in hand.

These concepts have been liberally proved by

Liberson and Magness. In fact, their original work (see the Bibliography at the back of the book) should be reviewed, if possible, as the results they obtained are quite impressive.

What does all this mean?

1. The biotonic exercises we recommend must be done every day.

2. A *maximal* effort to extend the joint, foot, knee, elbow, must be made but only to a count of six. With some exercises, even less.

3. They must be done daily for the magical twelve weeks; then as seldom as once a week to maintain full strength.

4. As your strength doubles so will your stamina, so you gain both ways.

5. Weights and other cumbersome apparatus are not necessary.

You will notice another thing as you read through the program: we recommend certain joint positions for certain exercises. This is because it is known that muscles develop more power in one position than in another. The muscles of the elbow joint, for instance develop most power when this joint is flexed at a ninety degree angle. So we have recommended that position for your elbow exercise. We have tried to find the best position for each joint but we give you a lot of leeway in choosing your own particular position for many of them.

Let's go back to the concept of stamina. We all want it, but how do we get it? As I have just said, stamina will increase as strength increases. But suppose one wants a *lot* of stamina, to run cross country, to row in competition, or to backpack in the mountains. How does one acquire this capability?

First, we must build strength. Then we can start with stamina training, for stamina demands a different muscle situation than does strength. For stamina, the blood supply must increase to bring new oxygen to the muscle and to remove the waste products. This means the heart must pump more blood. Improvement in storage of necessary components must take place. And the individual must learn tolerance to the pain involved in the activity, which is a gradual acclimation of the brain.

One idea you should clearly understand before you start is the law of individuality; each person is different. Don't give up your biotonics just because you can't be as strong as your neighbor, and don't gloat if you are stronger. I know it sounds like heresy to state that every person is not equal. I mean no challenge to the Constitution or the Law of God when I insist that muscle coordination and power in each of us is limited to our inherent capabilities. If everyone trained equally from the age of five, every day, and even ate the same food and had the same occupation, certain individuals would still emerge who could physically outperform everyone else with ease. The exercises in my biotonic program will not enable you to get in the ring with Muhammad Ali. At least, not for long.

Will they make you stronger, and build up your stamina and endurance? Yes, emphatically *yes!* If you are consistent and determined, I guarantee it. Remember, muscle strength is achieved as one would gain the top of a steep hill. You climb for a long while, wearily, becoming tired, almost quitting, and then, finally, you gain the top. With great ease you can now walk all over that hill. When you start your exercises, you will do fairly well for a short while, just like climbing the hill. After a day or so, your muscles will hurt a bit and they'll seem to lose strength. You'll be tempted to lay off, and you could go backward very rapidly. It will become very easy to say "To hell with it!" and quit.

But if you persist for the golden twelve weeks suggested by Dr. Mueller, you will suddenly see the light at the end of the tunnel. You will achieve your goal. After only three months, you will be trimmer, stronger, more confident and have more energy at the end of the day. Your biceps, stomach, legs—everything—will be firmer, healthier. Even after two months, you will feel like a totally new person.

While we are not interested in a "body beautiful" program, per se, your muscle size *will* grow with your strength and stamina (except if you're a woman, which I'll explain later). Increase in fiber size and blood supply will increase the muscle size. Charles Atlas looked so good because he had the capability for a certain size of muscle and developed that capability to full capacity. Thus we must take into account what we start with when we set our goals.

Figure 2 shows a chart listing the various types of individuals I had in mind when I developed this kind of biotonic exercise program. The chart applies to men and women. I have added a "housebody" section to apply to the individual who stays at home most of the time while his or her partner is off in the business world. Assuming this housebody will devote his or her home time to passive or active pursuits, I have generally categorized the housebody as either sedentary or active. The blue collar and white collar workers are categorized in three groups: sedentary, moderately active and active. Find yourself in the chart as closely as you can, according to your own evaluation of how active or inactive you are, your occupation, etc. Then determine your category and heed the instructions and warnings in the right-hand columns. When you are doing your exercises, take your category into consideration, and proceed accordingly.

You can see that the active blue collar worker's goals may be quite different from the white collar worker's. A man who works with his muscles all day long—shoveling, lifting, hammering, walking, pulling—will show it in his physical condition (unless he also overeats). Usually his legs will already be close to their inherent capacity in size and strength, and his back, belly and shoulders about the same. So, he may need two other things from the program: range of motion (ROM) for his joints, and exercise of the little-used muscles.

The cliché of the muscle-bound man is not a completely misleading one. Muscles can be enlarged until they press on nerves, blood vessels and yet other muscles, all of which tends to restrict joint motion. The range of motion exercises described in Chapter Four and delineated later in this book are designed to correct this, as well as to exercise the joints in the sedentary person. They will force the muscle to stretch and allow the joint its full range of motion.

But Blue Collar must remember that all of his muscles are not being equally exercised. Those being neglected depend upon his job, and he must analyze his own activity patterns and work on those that are slack. And he must remember at all times that we all tend to let our *gut* muscles

40

Figure 2

Self-Evaluation Chart for the Beginning Exerciser

Type	Exercise instructions
BLUE COLLAR	
Sedentary salesperson (stationary), assembly line worker, office worker.	Do ROM only for two weeks; then start the S&S exercises at a moderate pace.
Moderately Active waiter, mechanic, door-to-door salesperson, light duty truckdriver, police officer.	Do ROM only for one week; then start the S&S exercises at full contraction, 6-count.
Active longshoreman, firefighter, construction worker.	Proceed with ROM and S&S simultaneously; continue at own pace.
WHITE COLLAR	
Sedentary accountant, lawyer, banker, doctor, disk jockey, writer.	ROM only for three weeks; then start S&S moderately.
Moderately Active architect, surveyor, photographer, musician, artist.	Do ROM only for one week; then start S&S at own pace.
Active athletic coach, physical therapist, (there are few active white collar workers)	ROM only for four days; then start S&S at full contraction, 6-count.
HOUSEBODY	
Sedentary activities including reading, light housework, bookkeeping.	Do ROM only for one week; then start S&S at own pace.
Active active in leisure sports, heavy housework, gardening, home repair, caring for children.	Do ROM for four days; then start S&S at own pace.

slacken the most. We've all seen people with good builds, except for the oversized belly: the "beer belly" in the man with enormous shoulders and arms; the "potbelly" in the woman with an otherwise fine figure. This will be corrected by the belly-diaphragm and low-back exercises, done with special care. In the first month, for example, you will lose one inch at the waistline or else the exercises are not being done properly.

White Collar has a tough job ahead of him. About the only muscles that do much work in an office are the legs, and they do precious little. Pushing a pencil puts little demand on the rest of the body. Both range of motion and strength and stamina (S&S) work are needed in his exercises.

What can the average middle-aged white collar man expect from this biotonic exercise program? Several things. First, he can expect the circumference of his forearm and upper arm to increase one-half inch per month for three to four months and the circumference of his thighs about three-fourths inch.

Second, his muscle strength should show a dramatic increase—as much as forty percent the first month, and then level off to about ten percent per month for three months.

Third, he can expect, unless he is a thin man already, to lose from one to four inches from his waistline in two months.

Fourth, he can expect better posture almost immediately. Many of those little sharp muscle pains should leave. Aching and catching and burning miseries that sometimes hover around the back and shoulders, especially as we grow older, should disappear.

And last, while White Collar does not need reserve power and stamina to sit at his desk, he needs it for the weekend activities such as tennis, golf, handball, squash, running and swimming—even for cleaning out the attic or putting up wallboard. And he will have it. He will have it without paying the price of muscle pain or pulls. His muscles will be trim and held to the level of performance demanded by these exercises, and will easily meet the added demands for more strenuous work.

And what can a woman expect? Women and men are entirely different in their response to exercise and therefore we treat them separately. The male has testosterone; therefore, his muscles bunch and bulge and grow into great lumps. A woman's muscles do not. Hers become stronger, gain stamina but actually tend to thin a little as they strengthen. Women may expect to lose a half inch of circumference at their arms, perhaps three-quarters of an inch at the thigh and, depending on their shape when they start, several inches around the waist. Like the men, they can bid good-bye to those aching muscles after their occasional exertions.

But whether you are a woman or a man, you know what your requirements and weekend activities are better than I do. So set your goals and stick to them.

CHAPTER 3

Muscle Mechanics: Your Body as a Machine

This chapter is presented for those who, having made their decision to go on and persevere through the whole biotonic program, are curious to know in some physiological detail exactly what will happen to their muscles and joints over the next twelve weeks. It is, indeed, important to know what's going on with your muscles as you are exercising. I have found that being able to envision the motion of your bones, joints and muscles, makes it easier to exercise and actually mentally stimulates you into doing the exercises more meticulously.

Explanation is the balm of life. You can do anything better, go through any experience more easily with a little explaining. Every doctor knows this. The surgeon who sits down and talks to his patient before surgery and gives him the best idea possible about the operation, where the incision will be, what he will do inside, why he is doing it, what it feels like after surgery and what specific tasks the patient will have to do, this surgeon saves himself endless complications, and fewer lost tempers and emotional debauches. These exercises are no different. Do them, but also read what I say here and read what others say. If you can, get the original works I have listed at the back of this book and read them carefully. Study the anatomical drawings of your joint-muscles systems (See pages 47-51). The more you know, the more effective you become.

The very concept of biotonics is thought extension. You *think* of contracting the muscle, the muscle contracts. Thought—contraction. Every idea that helps the thought, helps the contraction. The more perfectly one understands the process of muscle-joint movement, the better one executes it.

However, I am not going to confuse the issue with puerile analogies of ropes and pulleys and chains and gasoline and tiny little men tugging on cords to contract something. Therefore, this short dissertation is semitechnical in nature, although by no means difficult for the layman to understand.

To begin with, you have to accept the disagreeable thought that your body is a machine, just a machine and nothing but a machine. You take in fuel in the form of food, burn it to supply energy to your body and perform such tasks (work) as will get you to the point at which you need more fuel (hunger). Wherein does this differ from the automobile that takes you to work?

Your machine is powered by muscles having exactly two actions and no more: contraction and relaxation. The contracting muscle force pulling

45

on two bones connected by a joint is the basic mechanism for body motion. Your bones are the levers of your body; your muscles pull them. These contractions are caused by nerve stimulation, which forces the muscle to contract just so much and no more. Thus you have *force* and *control*. The greatest muscle in your body can exert a force less than a gram to lift a pencil, or it can exert a force of hundreds of pounds to lift a great weight. In each case, the muscle exerts *exactly* enough force as is required of it to do the job, no more.

This control permits you to play a violent game of football, lift a child or fix a watch so fine you need a magnifier to see the wheels and gears. Whence comes this versatility?

All energy available to man came from the sun, until recently when he started drawing directly from the atom's core. But all the coal, gas, oil and plant energy on the earth is a direct storage of energy that began on the sun and, of course, came from the atom's core. The sun's rays work on all green plants through the magical substance called chlorophyll to produce plant food: carbohydrate, fat and protein. The plant absorbs compounds containing carbon, nitrogen and hydrogen and binds these together using this sun energy. Since it takes energy to make plant food, this food will release energy when it is burned in our bodies. That is what happens when wood burns in the fire—it simply releases sun energy stored in it during its manufacture. Similarly, the plant foods we eat release their energies (burn) in our bodies.

So we eat sun energy directly from green plants or indirectly from non-green plants or animals. All the energy from our food has three ultimate

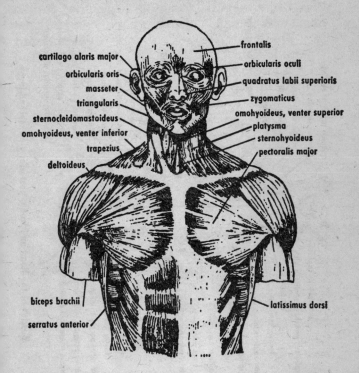

cartilago alaris major

orbicularis oris

masseter

triangularis

sternocleidomastoideus

omohyoideus, venter inferior

trapezius

deltoideus

frontalis

orbicularis oculi

quadratus labii superioris

zygomaticus

omohyoideus, venter superior

platysma

sternohyoideus

pectoralis major

biceps brachii

serratus anterior

latissimus dorsi

Muscles of the Head and Trunk, anterior view, first layer

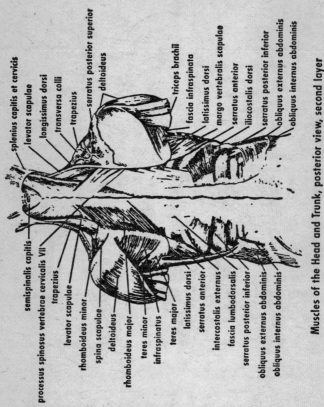

Muscles of the Head and Trunk, posterior view, second layer

Top labels (left to right):
semispinalis capitis
splenius capitis et cervicis
levator scapulae
longissimus dorsi
transversa colli
trapezius
serratus posterior superior
deltoideus
triceps brachii
fascia infraspinata
latissimus dorsi
margo vertebralis scapulae
serratus anterior
iliocostalis dorsi
serratus posterior inferior
obliquus externus abdominis
obliquus internus abdominis

Bottom labels (left to right):
semispinalis capitis
processus spinosus vertebrae cervicalis VII
trapezius
levator scapulae
rhomboideus minor
spina scapulae
deltoideus
rhomboideus major
teres minor
infraspinatus
teres major
latissimus dorsi
serratus anterior
intercostalis externus
fascia lumbodorsalis
serratus posterior inferior
obliquus externus abdominis
obliquus internus abdominis

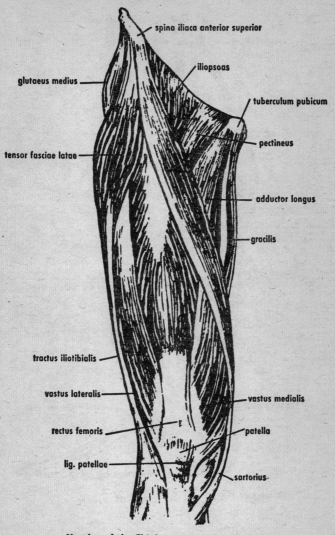

spina iliaca anterior superior

iliopsoas

glutaeus medius

tuberculum pubicum

pectineus

tensor fasciae latae

adductor longus

gracilis

tractus iliotibialis

vastus lateralis

vastus medialis

rectus femoris

patella

lig. patellae

sartorius

Muscles of the Thigh, anterior view, first layer

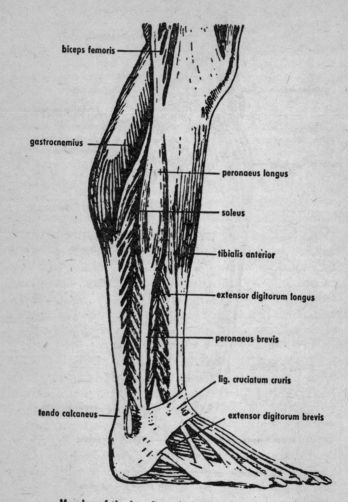

biceps femoris

gastrocnemius

peronaeus longus

soleus

tibialis anterior

extensor digitorum longus

peronaeus brevis

lig. cruciatum cruris

tendo calcaneus

extensor digitorum brevis

Muscles of the Leg, lateral view, first layer

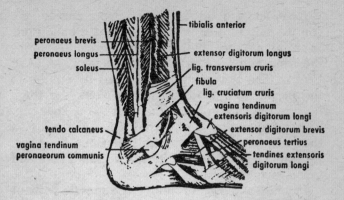

Foot, lateral view, showing the sheaths of the tendons

destinies: it is burned to produce body heat; it is burned to provide fuel for the metabolic activities—muscle motion, cell building, etc; or it is passed out of the body unused. An ideal life state for us would be one in which we take in the type and amount of food we need and use it completely: the steady state. Unfortunately, this rarely occurs. We more often get too much or too little food and food of the wrong kind.

Of the many metabolic activities necessary to the operation of the vastly complex human body, the one of interest to us here is the activity providing energy to our muscles. The muscles burn sugar, or chains of sugar, called glycogen. Any of the three basic food types—carbohydrate, fat and protein—can be changed to sugar in the liver and this sugar can be packed together into glycogen. The glycogen is carried to the muscles, where much of it is stored. When the muscles are contracted an immediate supply of glycogen or sugar is thus available.

Now, let's look at the muscle more closely. We can use any muscle in our body but a handy one to examine is the quadriceps, the muscle that forms the front and both sides of the thigh. Look at it. Feel it. The quadriceps is attached by tendon to the pelvic bone, and it extends along the thigh bone to the tendon that attaches it to the knee cap. This massive muscle of incredible power pulls on the knee cap tendon to straighten out the knee. As you can feel, the quadriceps is round, long and tapers toward the knee.

If you could look at your thigh muscle without the obscuring skin you would see it divided length-wise into sections about an inch in diameter. These sections are further divided by sheets of fine gristle. One can trace these divisions until he gets to the smallest division, the muscle fiber, or myofibril, itself. And here is where the action is.

This muscle fiber is just what its name says, a long, thin strand resembling a human hair in appearance. Its length is usually about the same as the muscle it serves, so the fibers in your thigh muscle are about two feet long. But they are only .01 to 0.1 mm in diameter. This long, thin organ does the muscle's work. It contracts like a self-powered rubber band to pull the tendons together, and these tendons make the bones move together on the joints. Motion is produced.

The microstructure of the muscle fiber has only recently come to be understood. It is a study in cooperation of many small things. Each fiber is but a long string of tiny little engines called sarcomeres which get shorter on command of their nerve. When all the sarcomeres along a fiber contract at once, each controlling only a few microns or so of shortening, the result is that the entire fiber contracts by one or two inches. And this is plenty to move the joint through its full range.

Of course each fiber is puny, but a million fibers and more acting together generate very great tension. A muscle can generate forty pounds per square inch of its cross-section.

The sarcomeres are strung together inside the muscle fiber like a string of square beads. And each sarcomere is rigidly joined to the one on either side of it. When a sarcomere contracts it pulls its two neighboring sarcomeres closer together. The "all or none" law governs all the sarcomeres in a fiber: either all of them contract or none of them do.

How does the brain control a mass of muscle fibers? This control stems from the way the muscle fibers and nerves are hooked together. Along the spinal cord lie a group of nerve bodies. Each sends its long axon through the femoral nerve, which springs out of the backbone, across the pelvis and into the leg, a distance of about three feet, to hook onto about one hundred muscle fibers in the quadriceps. These hundred fibers and the nerve are called the motor unit. When the brain sends an impulse down the spine and taps the nerve body, the hundred fibers are triggered into contraction by a denosine triphosphate (ATP). If this nerve is tapped repeatedly, as it is when the muscle is held rigid, then its hundred fibers are held in contraction. Only when the nerve stops sending impulses or when the fiber runs out of energy does the motor unit relax.

A hundred fibers seems a large number and all hundred have to fire together when the nerve says so—the "all or none law" again. This does not seem like very good control. But remember, there are thousands of groups of a hundred fibers each in this one muscle, thousands of motor units, and the brain can choose to fire only *one* group. *That* is control. The brain has a choice. It can stimulate one nerve and get a minimal response, several nerves for an intermediate response or all the nerves leading to this muscle for a maximal contraction.

Firing all at once, the nerves that lead to a muscle such as the quadriceps can bring about such a terrible contraction that the muscle may even be torn. *That* is power.

The brain may be thought of as a master pianist with millions of keys on its delicate instrument. It learns to press each key at the proper moment to bring about the proper response. The more it practices, the more perfect the response.

We all realize the muscle will change with repeated exercise. It enlarges and becomes stronger. The enlargement is due to increase in fiber size. Each fiber gains in diameter and probably in structural components such as actin and myosin. If one exercises daily with one hundred pounds, the muscles will enlarge until the required exercises may be done easily, then they get no larger unless more weight is used. Sports requiring many repetitions, like rowing, increase the muscles' blood supply as well as size.

The exercises you will be encouraged to do later will increase your muscle size. If these are done regularly with increasing force the muscle can be made quite large—in men. Not in women. Male testosterone is the reason for muscle enlargement. Women may become very strong but will *not* develop bulging muscles. So don't worry, ladies. Do your exercises and don't be afraid of acquiring "ugly" muscles.

CHAPTER 4

Range of Motion:
Importance of Healthy Joints

No one can "get in shape" without healthy joints. I don't have to draw diagrams to emphasize that without your joints you wouldn't be able to move at all, and that unhealthy joints are the causes of more ailments and afflictions of the human body than we care to acknowledge; certainly the cause of more pain. Most of us know someone with symptomatic arthritis or rheumatism, and we can see how much pain they have, how severely their joint motions are restricted, how "crippled up" they are. Words cannot describe the nausea and the strength destruction of joint pain, and *everyone* over forty has arthritis to some extent.

Therefore, no worthwhile exercise program can ignore the importance of healthy joints, nor can it exclude exercises especially for the joints—for maintaining the smooth, full motion of those joints as you go about your daily activities.

Joints which cannot make their full range of motion restrict the motion of other parts of the body. This, in turn, restricts the exercise of the muscles in that part, which rapidly leads to flabby, flaccid and sometimes severely atrophied muscles and eventual total immobility.

Therefore, before we can get our muscles and our whole bodies into vigorous, dynamic shape, we must start with the joints to assure smooth, liquid motion during any activity.

Range of motion, or ROM, means exactly what it says: how far the motion of a joint can be carried under normal circumstances. It is the single Most Holy Doctrine for your muscle-joint system, and the simplest. The one thing all your joints have in common is their need to be put through the full range of motion regularly in order to function properly—to balance the muscle pulls, the ligament pressures. You should work every joint of your body to its fullest extent at least three times a day.

Anatomically, a joint is that region where two or more rigid elements of the skeleton meet. In your arm, for example, where the forearm (the radius and ulna bones) meets the upper arm (the humerus), you have a joint called your elbow. If this joint fails to work properly (and it only "hinges" in one direction, if you'll note), or fails to work at all, you would be possessed of two rigid arms unable to bend. Consider for a moment the impact of such an affliction—how many functions do you perform wherein you are required to bring your hand in proximity to your face and head? How would you get along without that ability?

Similarly, your knee is the joint which allows your thigh bone (the femur) to hinge with your lower leg (the tibia and fibula). It, too, hinges in only one direction, and permits you to walk. Consider, again, where you would be without that "hinging" effect of the knee joint. Your wrists, your shoulders, your knuckles, your ankles, your spine, your hip are all vitally important joints which function smoothly and fluidly to allow you to perform certain tasks at work or play. Imagine an inflammation in those joints. Have you ever experienced the pain of trying to move a joint that refused to work properly, that wasn't lubricated adequately? The analogy of the rusty hinge isn't too far wrong.

Joints are usually classified in three groups: the synarthroses, which are immovable; the amphiarthroses, which are limited in their motion; and diarthroses, which are freely movable. The synarthrosis is actually a direct bony connection, except for an extremely thin layer of connective tissue or cartilage between the two bones. The skull is a good example. We've all seen depictions of the "plates" of the skull where cracklike sutures can be seen between plates of bone. For this exercise program, we can forget this kind of joint.

The amphiarthroses, or limited motion joints, have a fibrocartilage disk or plate between the two bony elements forming the joint. The bones may also be connected by a tough, inelastic ligament. The first kind of amphiarthrosis is found where the spinal vertebrae are joined with a disk (bend backward and you'll understand the "limited" motion concept). The second kind can be found where the upper ends of the tibia and fibula come together in your shin bone. While only a few of the ROM exercises are specifically aimed at the amphiarthroses, these joints will be more than adequately exercised just by running the other joints through their ROM.

By far the commonest joints, and those which will receive most of our attention, are the last in our list, the diarthroses. In this type of joint the bony elements being joined are covered by an articular cartilage and the joint itself is enclosed in a fibrous connective tissue capsule lined with a synovial membrane. This membrane produces a lubricating fluid which eases the motion of the joint, making it more freely movable. Without this fluid, raising your arm would be like rubbing two pieces of sandpaper together and the pain would be excruciating. I repeat this concept of pain and immobility to underscore the importance of smoothly movable joints to good health and stamina. When the joints begin to go, even though your muscles may be at top performance, you must give up the game.

There are several types of diarthroses, and you'll readily recognize them in your body. They are similar to machine parts, and some are named descriptively. There is the hinge joint, of course, such as your elbow and knee. Then there's the pivot type of joint; the ball-and-socket joint; the gliding joint; the saddle joint; and the ever-popular condyloid joint.

The hinge joint is further illustrated by the distal joints of the fingers. They move in one plane only, backward and forward. The jaw is also a hinge joint, although it also has some gliding motion. The knee and ankle joints are not typical hinges, since they also rotate, but they are essentially hinge joints.

A good example of one kind of pivot joint is the joint at the base of your skull between your first and second cervical vertebrae, the atlas and the axis. A protuberance from your axis, the second vertebra, inserts into the ringlike atlas, the first vertebra, and, with the two held in place by rigid ligaments, a rotating motion is permitted, such as shaking your head "no." Not to be morbid, but in death by hanging the ligaments are broken and the protuberance from the axis crushes the top of the spinal cord. In a word, these ligaments are *important!* Your elbow, where the radius and ulna are joined to the humerus, is an example of another kind of pivotal joint, wherein the radius is permitted to rotate.

The ball-and-socket joint permits the greatest range of motion and should receive the fullest attention when doing these exercises. This kind of joint allows rotation and flexion in a conical range limited in size only by the size of the two bones and the ligaments that join them together. Your hip and your shoulders are ball-and-socket joints —they are extremely important in work and athletic activities.

The joint is essentially just what it says it is: a ball inserted into a socketlike cavity, exactly like the universal joint on the axles of your automobile. The importance of exercising this kind of joint, and of assuring the required lubrication, cannot be overemphasized.

Your ankles and wrists are called gliding as well as hinge joints because they consist of two flat bones moving upon one another. Like many joints, they have a compound motion. The motion of all joints is limited by ligaments or by bony formations at the ends of certain bones.

The saddle-shaped joint is also self-descriptive. Picture a horseman in the saddle, able to move forward and backward or from side to side, but not both—he cannot rotate. That is, he cannot rotate without lifting himself off the saddle. This kind of joint is at the base of your thumb; a dislocation occurs when the thumb, the "horseman," is lifted off the saddle.

The condyloid joint is also characterized by the wrist joint, but that's enough medical jargon for now. Suffice it to say that you are now reasonably familiar with the types of joints in your body.

Fortunately (or unfortunately, depending on how old you are), babies exercise their joints better than adults do, which is one reason babies are usually healthier than adults. It is also why we grow up having any kind of joints at all. Babies run their joints through the full ROM almost instinctively. They flop and twist and stretch and bend like rubber mannikins, and their joints are marvelously fluid and free from pain. As we grow older, we neglect this vital action. That is, while we are forgetting to flop and twist and exercise those joints regularly, we are also forgetting how important it is to *do* them. We start to hold ourselves more and more rigid, keeping our arms and elbows at our sides, our heads straight ahead, letting our bellies sag outward and letting our spine bend the wrong way. Even the professional athlete, giving his all on the playing field, puts only a few of his joints through the full range of motion. That is why we *must* exercise our joints as well as our muscles if we are to gain strength and stamina.

Like every other gift, if we do not use our range of motion, we will lose it. The joints become less and less limber, the muscles more and more imbalanced, the joint capsule more tense. Finally, the lubrication stops, all motion stops and it becomes impossible to regain the lost motion.

Diseases and disorders of the joints are manifold. A weak joint can be easily dislocated, in which case there is displacement of one of the bones or a derangement of the parts that compose the joint. Once a joint is dislocated it is more easily dislocated in the future. Also the dislocation may possibly lead to loss of blood supply to the joint and joint destruction will then occur.

Bursitis is an inflammation of the bursal sac, a small, fluid-containing sac found under the skin that overlies pressure points. You have such bursas around your shoulders, knees, hips, etc. When these little sacs are irritated by friction or become inflamed they cause an aching pain.

There are two major and several minor types of arthritis. When I say everyone over forty has arthritis, I mean osteoarthritis, which is simply a wearing out process. All joints do this, possibly just from age itself. The rate at which the joints age from person to person is quite different and the amount of wear on particular joints is variable. The head-neck joint at the atlas creaks and grinds in all of us older types when we move our head back and forth (try it yourself if you are an older, over-forty type), while the shoulders set up quite a racket when the arm is turned through its full circle of motion. But the hips, knees and ankles usually stay smooth unless obesity is thrust on them. Osteoarthritis is the best argument for ROM exercises and for keeping the muscles firm, for it certainly develops more quickly and severely in abused joints.

The other major type of arthritis is rheumatoid.

61

This comes on as an acute inflammation. The joints swell and burn and get fiery red. The pain is sharp and excruciating. What causes this has long been debated with little success. It may actually be an infection caused by an organism too wily for our lenses or it may be an acute allergy—even to something in the body itself. Treatment regimens vary with the experts, as nothing has been found to cure the disease and preventing the disability of ruined joints is very difficult. While the acute inflammation is present, there is a tendency to put the joint at rest. Some therapists do use passive and active ROM exercises limiting the amount of motion to that tolerable to the patient. Certainly our ROM exercises can be used by such patients under the supervision of their therapist.

How many times have you sprained your ankle and heard:

"Oh, it's just a sprain. Nothing to worry about. Thank God, it's not broken!" And you extend your foot for the classic ankle strapping.

"Not broken, eh? Okay, kid, get out on that gridiron and give 'er hell. Best thing in the world for a sprain is a good workout."

Well, it is and it isn't.

It is true that the ankle can use the exercise while it is healing. It is not true that a "good workout" without proper support is the "best thing in the world for a sprain."

A sprain is *always* a tear in the ligaments. Around a finger, in the back, knee, but especially the ankle, ligaments are torn in a sprain. The patient steps wrong, the foot bends in and folds beneath him and the lateral ankle ligament is torn, the joint even temporarily dislocated. You can certainly see that the ligament is torn. The blue color beneath the skin is blood. Blood means torn blood vessels and the vessels were in that ligament. X-raying that ankle shows no broken bones, no attention is paid to the torn ligament and what happens? Before very long the same ankle is sprained again in precisely the same way.

Why? Because the lateral ligament that should be strong enough to keep the ankle from turning in has not healed from its first tear. Any little motion and another sprain is inevitable. This happened to me and before I met a man wise enough to put me in a cast I had sprained the same ankle *four* times. Six weeks in a cast worked a miracle. If you don't want your sprained ankle put in a cast, there are now braces available. These are canvas, have steel straps in the side to keep the ankle from turning in and yet let it move freely from front to back. But remember, ligaments heal at the same rate as bone. It takes six weeks, at least, to heal a ligament. Keep the cast or brace on for that time, at least.

I often wonder, when the "Oh, it's just a sprain" philosophy is bruited around, why we still fall for it. One of the greatest of all orthopedists, Sir Reginald Watson-Jones, devoted considerable space to this problem in his book *Fractures and Joint Injuries*, printed in 1955, and that was 22 years ago. Surely by now the precepts of this fine man should have filtered into all of our hands.

Sprains are one more good argument for static thrust power. The powerful muscles move to protect a joint under attack and may possibly prevent spraining.

Around every joint is a tough band of gristle called, as we said before, the joint capsule. Attached to this are ligaments and tendons which, together, limit the amount of motion expected from any given joint. If we examine the ROM of some joints, we find a great difference. The ankles, for example, move backward and forward only about 40 degrees and they turn inward approximately 20 degrees. The neck swivels a full 180 degrees and does almost as well bending forward and backward. But the shoulder—ah, that's the real marvel. The magnificent shoulder is so constructed that it can rotate in almost a complete circle.

But, the real marvel is also the real crybaby. While other joints cause pain when they lose ROM and hurt in varying degrees, the shoulder will not tolerate even the slightest loss of ROM. *If we do nothing but exercise this one joint, the shoulder, we will have saved ourselves a grinding ball of trouble!* The shoulder is probably one of the three most important joints in your body (the hip and the neck being the others), and certainly the one, with the hip and neck, which is most critical in athletic endeavors and heavy work. We will be paying much attention to the shoulder in our exercises.

Now you may say, "Is that all? Move my joints? Wiggle my arms and legs around? Sounds like sissy exercises to me!"

And you'd be right. In fact, I *call* them the "Sissy Exercises" for that very reason. They are simple, easy, take little effort and can be done almost anywhere, yet they are one of the most important sets of exercises the human body can perform. Too often, the "get-in-shapers" are working out, lifting weights, running, jogging, dieting, giving up smoking—whatever—and they are forgetting their joints. They become trim, if they're men their muscles bulge, but their joints are going downhill fast. They won't last the normal lifetime. I remember a case recently—*a* case?—good heavens, I can remember dozens of them. All my athletic friends. I beg, plead, even threaten to shut off the hot water to their showers but it does no good. They will *not* do ROM or static thrust exercises. They refuse even to lift their weights. But they will go and knock themselves out every lunch break on the handball courts. When I examine them in the office, I find shoulders that grind like coffee mills, knee joints like rough emery grit and ankles like carborundum.

"Are you getting warmed up before you exercise? Do you do your ROM and static thrust exercises?" I ask politely.

"Oh no, I don't do that. I've been jogging. Great for the legs." Or, "I've been swimming. Keeps me in shape for handball."

And so on and so forth.

As I said, I think the shoulder exercises are the most important ones I can offer. They will save you immense pain now and later.

Don't be like the rest of my patients. *Do your joint exercises religiously! Be the most supple one on your block!*

CHAPTER 5

Your Stomach or Your Health

The old routine Jack Benny used to pull might well apply to a lot of people who are continually overweight and sluggish. A thief approaches Jack, gun in hand, and commands: "Your money or your life!" Jack pauses, as the audience starts to chuckle. Finally, as the suspense gets too much to bear, the thief shouts impatiently: "Well? *Well?*" And Jack responds, "I'm *thinking*, I'm *thinking!*"

I suspect a lot of people would pull the same thing if a doctor commanded, "Your stomach or your health!" That is, I know a lot of people who would rather eat than exercise, and who don't understand that that attitude is going to kill them years before their time. Even as much as ten years!

There are a hundred *trillion* cells in your body. If you like to look at zeros, that's 100,000,000,000,000 cells, and each one is a vitally important building block in the system, the machine, that is your body. Each of these cells lives and dies, and is replaced by new cells which are manufactured by the food we eat. A cell can be healthy or unhealthy; impoverished or nourished, just as you yourself may feel. In fact, it's a good practice to consider yourself only as one of your cells. As *you* feel, so does each cell. If you are in good shape, physically and chemically, so is your cellular structure. "You are what you eat," "Food makes the man," and many other aphorisms concerning diet and nutrition are not only true, they are *absolutely* true. That is because we can function on the food we eat *only* if that food contains the necessary building materials and energy we need to build and feed our body cells. Everything you own—your muscles, your organs, your blood, your heart, your brain, eyes, teeth, tongue, toes—is composed of cells which need daily nutrition. They can only find this nutrition in what we put into our stomachs (and the oxygen we breathe). Therefore, if we are to build muscle strength, and achieve a higher degree of stamina and endurance for the rest of our lives, we must ingest only those foods which are good for us, and totally eliminate foods and chemicals which are bad for us.

Sound simple? It's not.

Anyone about to undertake an exercise program must take stock of what he is putting into his stomach. A person could quite literally grow fatter and fatter into obesity, even while exercising vigorously every day, because he is eating too much and eating the wrong foods. So let's investigate some basic components of food, and take a quick refresher course in nutrition. I know about all the fad diets, about the cholesterol scare, about calories and carbohydrates, the drinking man's diet, the Mayo clinic diet, the water diet and the no-salt diets. I'm going to tell you the *facts* about food and muscle conditioning and strength. I had been practicing medicine for twenty years before I finally appreciated the disastrous effects of ingesting refined sugar on the human body. Thank goodness, new studies are "refining" the woefully inadequate nutritional facts available when I was a student.

First, a word about our trusted, much abused friend, the stomach. No organ, including the heart, puts up with as much abuse and general negligence as the stomach. In the course of our lifetime we treat it simultaneously like a garbage pail, scapegoat, reservoir, whipping boy and laboratory rat. As children we throw enormous quantities of sugar and unknown substances into it. As teenagers we ask it to digest impossible substances like oils and greases and strange preservatives such as those in the fast and frozen foods. As adults we throw massive doses of alcohol into it before we think to prepare it with food for absorption. We worry and fret ourselves into ulcers and nervous disorders of the stomach. In fact, among the chief conditions of the stomach requiring surgery are ulcers, tumors and foreign substances—most of which are the product of our own behavior and not accidental. We put wild spices into our stomachs; hot sauces; bilious, gelatinous fluids; aspirins and foaming "cures"; we even eat live goldfish and light bulbs. There is a man in the Guinness Book of Records who systematically tried to eat a car!

Poor stomach. It sits there, taking all this abuse, trying desperately to do its job and prepare our food for digestion and subsequent transformation into life-giving, muscle-building nutrients. And, for the large part, it remains uncomplaining. Maybe an upset here and there, maybe it will regurgitate on you now and then, or it will gently remind you to let up for a while with a few well-timed belches and burps.

The stomach has two functions, usually serving them both with a minimum of fuss. It stores, mixes and prepares food, and it begins the digestive process. Actually starch digestion is begun in the mouth when it is attacked by the amylase in the saliva. But this has only a mild effect. The real digestive work takes place in the stomach, and this work starts even before food hits the stomach. Just the smell and sight of food starts the juices rolling. As a good steak calls out the saliva, so it calls out the gastric juice. When food hits the stomach there is waiting a green sea of digestive ferments: renin to curdle milk; pepsin to take apart proteins and break them into simpler compounds; lipase to chew up fat; and bunches of lesser enzymes. This sea is a bath of hot, strong hydrochloric acid that lets all these enzymes do their work.

Why such a complex process? The ultimate answer is because all food has to be broken down to its basic parts before we can use it. There exists in each of our bodies a template, a model, a master plan. By whatever name, this model judges everything that comes into our body. If we were to take a slug of pork chop, grind it up and inject it into our veins, it would kill us. Our bodies would recognize this as foreign material, gang up on it and set up such a reaction we would die. This same pork chop is as sweet in the mouth as wild honey and builds good muscle in the man. Why the difference between the reactions in the vein and in the mouth?

We know that protein is a complex and very specific chemical. Every human builds protein in a slightly different way. But the twenty amino acids that we use to build these proteins can be used just as they are by everybody. It is a bit like stealing building blocks from the Great Pyramid to build smaller temples.

So our bodies can absorb and use the amino acids, the building blocks, but the temples themselves have to be built according to the specifications of each body, according to its model or template. And that is the difference between the vein injections and eating the muscle; when eaten, the digestive enzymes work on the muscle and convert it to its component building blocks. The stomach does not break down every food, but the stomach begins the process, carrying out the toughest part, the initial part of tearing apart the protein and fat.

The stomach is hollow and muscular, a highly secretory organ located on the left side of your upper abdomen. It is *not* directly behind your belly button. If you put your index finger right below the last rib on your left side, and press inward gently, you'll be pointing directly at your stomach.

The stomach is shaped roughly like a J, and is connected at its upper end to the esophagus, or gullet. At the lower end it feeds directly into the small intestine via the pylorus, or pyloric valve. The upper portion of the small intestine, which receives food from the stomach first, is called the duodenum.

The size and shape of your stomach, not surprisingly, is considerably variable. Its volume goes from 1,000 to 1,500 cc normally, and the entrance to it is normally occupied by a small air bubble.

The walls of the stomach consist of four coats. The first or inner coat is a mucous membrane which contains numerous convoluted glands called rugae which secrete digestive enzymes and hydrochloric acid. The second coat consists of loose fibers, called submucosa, which contain nerves and blood and lymph vessels. The third coat is muscle, three layers of it. The fourth coat, the serosa, covers the greater part of the stomach and connects with the peritoneum, or the lining of your entire abdominal cavity.

The stomach has both a secretory and a motor function. The main reservoir for the food you've eaten is the fundus, the largest section of the stomach, where the gastric juice softens and saturates the food preparatory to its passage into the small intestine. Psychological factors may play an important part in the secretion of such gastric juice, however, which is why extreme grief, shock or other abnormal mental attitudes have such an impact on digestion and stomach activity. (See Chapter Seven, the Psychology of Exercise.) The motor function of the stomach consists of peristaltic action in which the lining of the stomach churns and "mashes" the food into a mushy substance, which is transferred in very small portions to the small intestine.

It should be easy now to see what happens when we stuff ourselves at the dinner table. There is only so much volume our stomachs can accommodate, and when we exceed that volume the stomach has to stretch itself to handle the new volumes of food. Hence, we may find ourselves having to eat more and more to satiate the feeling of hunger, brought about by the greater volume of the stretched stomach. This in turn forces us to eat more (since we seem to be too weak to push our-selves away from the table). Also, when the stomach is stuffed beyond its capacity, food being sent to the small intestine for ultimate digestion may not be as adequately prepared by gastric juice as it should be. This in turn puts an added burden on the intestines and other parts of the digestive tract.

In other words, no good can ever come from overeating! Even a starving man rescued from the desert, or a horribly undernourished prisoner of war, cannot be stuffed with food to overcome the deficiencies. The digestion of food and the nourishment of the cells thereafter takes place at its own rate—higher volumes of food do not speed digestion!

But in America we are not trying to speed digestion. We are trying to slow it down. America wallows in a food glut that makes the seven good years of Joseph's Egypt look like a weenie roast. We have stored up the vastest food stores that ever were gathered. The finest technology to festoon this planet makes the entire operation of planting, weeding, bug proofing, harvesting, preparing and delivering food completely automatic. Like the enchanted buckets the Sorcerer's Apprentice set in motion, we have set our food machine in motion and cannot stop it. We have food, food, food—and that food is *energy*.

This food falls into three types: carbohydrate, fat and protein. Each has its special function, and each should be considered in a brand new light during my biotonic exercise program. Each predominates in certain foods. Carbohydrate is essentially sugar. There are various kinds, such as glucose, fructose, galactose, sucrose, but they all break down to and are burned as glucose. So all sugar foods—cake, ice cream, sweet rolls, candy, honey, all starches such as potatoes and beans, all fruits and sweet vegetables—contain carbohydrates.

Fats are obvious. All greasy foods contain fats. Most fats are found in meats; deep fried foods are drenched in fat.

Important proteins are found in the animal and vegetable world. All meat—the muscle of edible animals—fish, poultry, eggs, are high in animal proteins. And these are very good proteins and easily assimilated by the young child. Legumes—peas, beans, soybeans, peanuts—nuts and all grains are high in vegetable protein.

Milk is high in all three types of food. Its whey is almost pure protein and from this we get cheese, which is a concentrated source of protein.

Carbohydrate is the delicate food of the fastidious brain and provides energy to the rest of the body. That's all, just energy. The sugar molecule is eaten, absorbed across the lining of the small intestine and shunted into the bloodstream almost immediately. (This, by the way, is why one gets drunk quickly on an empty stomach—the alcohol molecule is passed directly to the small intestine, where it enters the bloodstream instantly, with no digestion required.)

In the blood, the sugar molecule may be stored or used immediately. If used, it is broken down by low energy transfer processes until its residue becomes water and carbon dioxide gas, and is passed out of the body via the lungs and the urinary tract.

In the process of being used, or even merely circulating in the bloodstream, sugar forces the pancreas to react. And the pancreas secretes insulin. This chemical allows the sugar to be used by the cells or stored in the liver. However, the pancreas is not a very discriminating organ. A large bolt of sugar makes it overshoot its mark and secrete too much insulin, which causes the blood sugar level to fall much lower than is good for your disposition. My name for this condition is "sugar shock." The pancreas is a highly overreacting organ, and should be pampered. More on this later.

Fat is a dull, sludgy substance that makes nice curves in the proper amounts. Too much and it turns you into a modified sausage, both internally and externally. And the one thing you can say for fat, brother, is that *it sticks with you.* Boy, is it loyal! Once fat has accumulated in the human body, one must work like hell to get it off. It makes eminently better sense to keep it off in the first place than to "get in shape" after you've acquired what you think is too much of it. And if you're over forty, once you've achieved the conditioning you want from this program, stay there! It becomes progressively more difficult to take off fat as you get older.

Another thing you can say about fat: it's high in calories. (Are you getting the feeling that fat is one of your true enemies?) No food can approach fat for energy, which is what calories are all about. One can easily store enough fat to provide himself with enough calories for months of free living. Eskimos do it out of necessity, Americans do it out of sloth.

Counting calories is the hot gimmick of the "fad" dieter. Unfortunately, he rarely knows what a calorie is and he neglects other important aspects of his diet.

"Yeah, I had a good lunch," he says. "I cut out the roast beef and the vegetables and that gave me almost two hundred extra calories and then I could have a piece of lemon meringue pie."

Counting calories will make you slimmer, there is no doubt about that. If you take in fewer calories than you burn up, you will lose weight. You are forced to burn your own body stores: first, sugar, then fat and then protein. Getting to the point at which you burn body protein takes immense persistence and is not something one need worry about very much.

Unfortunately, counting calories is curing the symptoms and not the disease. As soon as you stop counting your calories, you're going right back where you were at the beginning: overweight. This is because your basic diet and exercise routine was all wrong to begin with. It is sad that the calorie has become the mythic god of diet.

A calorie is merely the amount of energy required to raise one cubic centimeter of water one degree centigrade. That's all it is, a unit of heat. It's not a "thing," something you could look at under a microscope. It is the heat you get from burning a certain amount of a certain food. And this energy can go to fuel the body functions, or it can be stored as fat. Just remember, it *has* to go some place.

So counting calories is not important: the important thing is the foods themselves. The danger is that counting calories could lead you to rule out many very nutritious foods that are high in calories in favor of better tasting but far less nutritious foods.

Okay, I've attacked the mythic god and opened this whole confusing subject, so let's go all out and get down to a few facts on nutrition that make some sense.

To start with, why is nutrition so complex? Why do we hear something different from every authority in the land, from Congress to the dietician at Podunk Center? Is it really this confusing? Yes, it is, for two reasons. First, there are literally thousands of natural foods in the world. Almost every kind of life from bacteria to man himself has been used as food by man and each of those foods has certain nutritional characteristics. So we can meet our food needs with an infinite number of food combinations.

Second, modern technology has increasingly altered our food; it has "refined" it. Now here is a nasty term, and before we are finished with this subject I hope "refined" will be the dirtiest word in your nutrition vocabulary. Refined food is degraded food. The more refined it is, the less food value it has. If I attack "sugar" I am attacking *refined* sugar, not natural sugar; *refined* sugar shorn of its natural vitamins, minerals and proteins.

But, get this straight. I do not attack, nor indict, nor glance with any disparagement on the refiners, the manufacturers or purveyors of refined foods. These people exist because we, the eaters, demand that there *be* refined foods. We think they taste better. They are daintier.

Before we refined food, nutrition *was* simple.

Our ancient ancestor killed animals and ate them whole, grew grain and ate that whole, drank whole milk and ate whole eggs and gathered fresh vegetables which he ate whole. And he flourished. The best of all foods are those of animal origin and especially those which nature has provided for the nourishment of the growing animal. Our ancester took in the perfect proteins: the lactalbumin and casein of milk, ovitellin and albumin in eggs, the meat and wheat and soybean and maize proteins. All these perfect proteins built of all twenty

76

essential amino acids he took in every day in whole-sale quantities. He had power, stamina, vitality. His cheeks burned with good health, his body was inexhaustible. Women bore straight, strong babies and they fed these babies also on whole grains, meat, cheese, nuts and milk.

The human race simply cannot stand prosperity. In Roman times we read how the patricians demanded refined food and refined wines. Pliny warned them. Their refined wines contained lead, deadly poison that killed them like flies. When an army of these patricians met the army of Julius Caesar on the plains of Pharsalia, they were massacred like sheep. They, with their refined foods and dainty wines, were insignificant straws against Caesar's flaming warriors who ate whole grains and meat.

Therefore, the real answer to "Why is nutrition so complex?" is *because refining foods makes it so.*

As a machine, your body has certain energy needs that must be met by food. This energy goes to move the body or to rebuild it. If the body is to maintain the same weight, it must take in as much energy as it uses, and no more. Thus, the law of conservation is served in your body as it is everywhere else in the universe. This law allows us to make two statements: if the body takes in more energy than it uses, it must increase its weight; if less energy, it must decrease its weight.

Everybody on this planet, all four billion of us, has a different energy requirement, so we all must eat a little differently. Our energy requirements depend on age, sex, race, climate, habits, our ability to digest and absorb food and our ability to metabolize or burn it. Not only are these energy requirements variable from person to person but they vary for the same person at different times. How do we ever judge our food intake?

Fortunately, most of us are equipped with a highly specialized area in the ancient part of our brain called the hypothalamus. I call this ancient because animals living 400 million years ago had well developed hypothalamuses and ours are no different from theirs. This specialized area is called the "appestat." Obviously, the word is a cross between "appetite" and "stat" and means "to stabilize the appetite." This appestat tells us by hunger pains, weakness and other symptoms, when and how much we should eat. If we listen to it carefully and do not let our desires, fears, angers, greeds or hates overcome us, it will accurately hold a perfect weight for us.

Unfortunately, about a million factors clobber our ability to listen to our appestats. We don't like this food or that. We have to have refined food. Our mothers teach us that this food is good, that one is bad, etc., etc. So, the appestat becomes an unreliable guide. Either it has us eat too little, as those rare, rare people who hate food do, or it has us eat too much, as all the rest of us do.

The vast majority of Americans are not able to rely on the appestat. Our instincts are completely useless. Only our intellects can direct our food consumption to the maximal benefit of our bodies. Certainly, primitive man, that fabulous ancestor, could rely on his appestat; but we cannot. We must rely on our intellects to select our modern American diet and for this we need facts.

Starting with carbohydrate, we ask, need we eat sugar? The answer is, no. We need eat no sugar, nor any food to which sugar is added. No cakes, pastries, sweet rolls.

78

"But," you scream, "my brain needs sugar. How can I *think* without sugar?"

Easily. Your body can efficiently make all the sugar your brain needs from protein and fat. You need never add sugar to your diet again if you get enough protein. We have already told you how sugar stirs up one's insulin and we'll describe this in more detail, but this is not its only undesirable trait. Sugar spares protein and fat.

It does this by being easily burned. In a hearth fire the little twigs burn quickly and the logs slowly. The same is true with burning fat and protein versus sugar. When the body burns sugar, it does not go through the laborious process of burning the protein by converting it down to urea, nor burning the fat. Instead it stores the fat in deposits that make the hips bulge. Again, as the little twigs burn quickly, so the carbohydrate is gone soon after it is eaten and again hunger is gnawing at our bellies.

Everyone damns fat. Obviously, for it destroys the American's idea of beauty. But fat alone will not make us fat. If we eat no carbohydrate, the body cannot store this fat. It is carbohydrate and not fat that destroys our curves. This is not to indict the carbohydrates occurring naturally in balanced proportions in fruits and vegetables. Certainly these excellent foods are to be taken in moderation. But let us not add refined sugar, that super-sweetener, to our diet, either as sugar per se or as products made sweet with it. This is the carbohydrate that makes all of America a vast Fat City.

And fat is not all bad. Fat is the great cushioner and insulator in the body. Every delicate organ is surrounded by fat, cushioned, protected and held in place by fat. We walk on the fat of our soles and grasp with the fat of our palms and yearn for the fat of her curves. And we draw on this fat in times of need. Only in excess is fat harmful.

It is not fat in general that sends the doctors to their typewriters to report human-saving advances, but specifically *saturated* fat. This is the alleged bad guy that fouls up the blood vessels and makes us old before our time. Saturated and the worst, the very worst of all—cholesterol! According to common belief, here is another dirty word. But I said there would be only one dirty word; so I am about to take up the cause of cholesterol and lay before you the defense of the egg.

Why is cholesterol supposed to be so terrible? It suffers from guilt by association. Whenever hardening of the arteries exists, termed atherosclerosis by medical men, there we find cholesterol.

You pick up a boiled egg, salt it, but before you get it to your mouth you think, "My gosh, man, you're not going to eat that, are you?"

You look at the innocent oval as your inner voice continues in horror, "That contains *cholesterol!*"

And you set that egg down as if it were an ugly bug. "Cholesterol," you think, "and I almost ate it!"

I am frequently asked about diet by my patients and when I admit to eating *two* eggs a day they look at me as if *I* were an ugly bug.

"What do *you* do for breakfast?" I will ask.

Invariably they tell me they either eat none at all or they have a "roll and coffee" and always in a tone that indicates that they would rather die than touch an egg and "all that cholesterol."

So, to get some sense into diet we must wrestle with cholesterol. And we have to fight with the knowledge that what we say today may be disproved tomorrow.

No one can deny the ugly plaques along our arteries that clog off the blood flow to our hearts and brains, and no one can deny these plaques contain large amounts of cholesterol. This is a fact. When one opens an artery to a heart dead of a "coronary" or heart attack, he sees thick, sludgy fat laced with sharp calcium choking the lifeblood out of the heart. We must admit cholesterol is always at the scene of the crime. But, after all, so are the police. Are we condemning a true friend when we refuse to eat cholesterol?

Consider. Cholesterol is a very complex molecule with five rings of carbon atoms and several side chains, about as complex as a fine watch. Yet our bodies can build this molecule from scratch. Taking the little two-carbon acetate molecules, it strings these together like a kid with an Erector Set until it has put this complicated molecule together. Why does the body and specifically the lining of the blood vessels—the very point where we are most vulnerable to cholesterol—have this remarkable ability? Is it because we are constructed to self-destruct?

Consider further. Atherosclerosis occurs almost exclusively in the arteries where the high pressure and high strains exist. It worsens with increasing blood pressure which further strains the artery, and it always occurs at the point of greatest stress. We can predict the sites of formation of atherosclerotic plaques in the arterial walls with deadly accuracy, and these predictions are made on a knowledge of hemodynamic flow principles. The plaques always occur at the points of greatest stress. Does it seem reasonable that *only* those areas of the artery wall where strain will exist because of blood flow will be able to make cholesterol? Does it not seem more likely that cholesterol is laid down as a cushioning material to protect against the hydraulic ram of that pounding blood?

Another point. Damage to the arterial wall leads to atherosclerosis. Crushing, hitting, cutting the artery all set up these cholesterol plaques! Does the body do this to destroy any of its arteries that are hurt or is this part of the general process of repair, an attempt to protect that part of the artery?

And yet another point. The amount of cholesterol circulating in the blood at any particular moment can be raised by stimulating the hypothalamus. Here is our friend, the hypothalamus, again. This area of the brain has almost endless responsibilities to regulate the amount of the blood substances. In health it always regulates these substances in such a way as to protect the body and assure its survival. Yet, here it is increasing the blood cholesterol, which is presumably dangerous.

We know stress is bad for us. Whether it be the stress of being beaten up, of being angry, a job we hate, driving fifty miles to work each day, an all-night dance or poker game or our neighbor's dog barking till dawn, it is bad for us. It strains our bodies, raises blood pressure, interferes with sleep. In short, it places us under stress and that is bad. And these stresses all increase the blood cholesterol by acting on the hypothalamus.

Type A and Type B coronary risks have become newsworthy. The Type A patient is hard-driving, aggressive, fighting for his job and the things his job will buy by beating out his competitors. Type B is much more complaisant. Type A gets the heart attack, Type B does not. Type A is obviously under stress as we know it. He generates more adrenalin (the fight-or-flight hormone), more cortisone (the great hormone that always works to balance the body) and he makes more cholesterol, much more than Type B.

Now, it would be absurd to say that cholesterol in the blood *causes* stress. All the evidence is that stress increases the blood cholesterol. Since stress causes the body to make more adrenalin, cortisone and other substances that help it tolerate the stress, why would the cholesterol be increased to destroy the body during stress?

When we further note that cholesterol is the molecule that cortisone comes from, that without cholesterol the body cannot make the absolutely vital and necessary cortisone, it seems again that cholesterol is more a friend than a killer.

Lastly, why single out cholesterol? Recent work shows smoking is a major cause of atherosclerosis, probably through increasing the level of carbon monoxide in the blood. This is quite well proved in several ways. Even damage to the heart muscle itself has been produced in the experimental animal that is exposed to smoke. Blood pressure alone has a powerful effect on atherosclerosis and heart attacks; both of these increase in proportion to the pressure. In addition, various trace elements, those necessary only in tiny amounts in our bodies, are shown to be involved in atherosclerosis. Chromium seems to exert a protective effect and cadmium a destructive effect on the blood vessels. And it is rather clear that *refined* sugar *raises* the blood cholesterol and, by implication, is conducive to hardening of the arteries.

When we put all this evidence together with the bank of other variables that enter into the study of heart disease, variables like age, sex, race, diet, climate and occupation, it becomes pretty obvious that cholesterol is but one of many enigmas in the disease. Perhaps it does not deserve to be singled out as the culprit.

One more point and we will let our defense of the egg rest. There are certain substances that enhance or increase the excretion of fats. Chief among these is choline. It is a simple compound, compared to cholesterol, but extremely important. It prevents overaccumulation of fats of all kinds in the liver. One needs choline to keep his liver from suffocation in fat. Choline is found in meat, kidney, liver—up to 600 milligrams per hundred grams of these tissues. But the egg! It has from 1,400 to 1,700 milligrams, that is, from 1.4 grams to 1.7 grams of choline per hundred grams of yolk. The egg has a built-in fat controller surpassing anything else available to us, yet we refuse to eat eggs because they contain cholesterol. Hardly makes sense, does it?

In this day of the return to nature and emphasis on natural foods, it would seem unnecessary to write the above argument. Nature knows best and what is natural and unrefined is better. After all, nature has had some 500 million years of practice while we have been at it for only the last hundred or so.

If we have thoroughly defended the egg, we can discuss the third basic food, protein. To modern Americans, protein is critically important. It has about all we need and several cagey little characteristics besides that go along with jet age life. As we said, our problem is too much weight, and protein is our best ally. You skinny exercisers can eat all the carbohydrate you want but the rest of us better read carefully what I say about protein.

We can live on protein. It contains amino acids

which can be built up to other products as needed by the body and it has the nice characteristic of not being stored. If we eat more protein than we need, the excess is passed off harmlessly. The excess protein is excreted largely in the bowel. The kidneys have no problem secreting nitrogen, so they are not overloaded. Indeed, protein is the base of uric acid which causes the gout we mentioned in Chapter One, but only if you have a genetic predisposition to the disease need it concern you. Such a tendency may easily be checked by a blood test.

But, while protein can substitute for carbohydrate and fat, the reverse is not true. There is no way to build the twenty essential amino acids in the human body. These have to be taken in with the diet in daily amounts, cannot be stored but are used as eaten or passed off. We can live on protein but not on fat or carbohydrate.

Protein helps us lose weight. Each of our three basic foods increases the heat production in the body when eaten. Fat increases heat four percent, carbohydrate six percent, but protein snaps it up a whopping thirty percent. Just eating protein, therefore, fires off more heat and helps burn excess fat. And protein is not completely burned. Carbohydrate and fat are burned completely, all the energy is drained out to be kept in the body. Not protein. At the most, only sixty percent of its energy is gotten out as it is burned down to urea, which is excreted in the urine. In addition, it costs the body energy to build proteins from amino acids. If no carbohydrate is eaten, this energy has to come from the body and the fat stores are depleted. Thus a high protein diet has several ways of taking off weight.

"But," you might object, "I can't eat protein without eating fat. Every meat contains fat and some meats have a lot of it." That is correct, but this fat is of no concern. Protein alone will not provide enough energy to store this fat, nor will the fat burn the protein. Therefore, this combination will not increase your weight. As you increase your protein intake your body will store it for a few days, but then it will adapt to the new load and excrete the excess.

Now, there are two obvious disadvantages to the high protein diet: it is not satisfying and it can be carried to extremes. I do not advise the extremes. I lay down some facts to be used carefully so the moderate person may lose weight wisely and hold his optimum level. Your doctor will tell you what weight you should reduce to and the moment you reach it, add starches and other natural but more fattening foods to your diet. If you follow a diet of whole cereal grains, legumes, milk, meat, eggs and cheese, you will automatically balance your diet for this will supply some natural carbohydrate.

But remember, a high protein diet feels like starvation, especially at the beginning when your body feels the withdrawal symptoms of no sugar. You are always as hungry as if you were fasting and you are almost as weak. Protein does not satisfy hunger quickly. It is absorbed slowly from the small bowel and never gets the blood sugar up high enough to turn off the appestat. You won't have those terrible shaking depressions and manias of sugar shock that follow a binge of sugar intake, but you won't have that hour or so of total contentment that follows eating a sweet roll either.

Instead of the roller coaster of depression and

mania, you totter along in a steady gray state of not feeling really good but not feeling really bad, either. You strike a mean between your peaks and your valleys. But you are burning excess fat, feeding your muscles the proteins they need both for energy and for repair and assuring yourself of a constant supply of all essential amino acids.

If you enjoy being fat, crammed into your body, bulging your britches and popping out of your shirts and blouses, by all means keep up a high sugar intake. But if the derisive stares of your friends and spouse are more painful than you can bear, then take up the pain of this high protein diet. One way or another you have to take pain; choose which is worse.

The fourth type of food substance, and as controversial as sin itself, is vitamins. What to believe? One source tells you that your body desperately needs them, and another says it's a lot of bunk. We prefer not to get embroiled in this little tempest, leaving the subject to the greats like Linus Pauling. However, over my many years of surgical practice, I have noticed that one basic rule might apply, and I recommended it to those entering into my exercise program. And this is, *you've got nothing to lose and lots to gain by taking a daily vitamin supplement.*

The truth of the matter cannot be much simpler:

1. Food cannot be adequately burned without vitamins.

2. A lot of the food Americans eat is vitamin deficient.

3. We often overcook food, destroying vitamin value.

4. The body eliminates vitamins it doesn't need.

Ergo, the Wiederanders Conclusion: Take a good vitamin supplement daily, even if you think your diet is adequately balanced. What have you got to lose?

Now, keeping in mind this brief review of Home Ec 101A, what does the person who wants to get in shape do to maintain a good diet?

After you take your vitamin (actually it should be taken after there is already some food in the stomach), eat a good protein breakfast. I cannot emphasize this enough—a good *protein* breakfast. The exact form is up to you, but I'll make some suggestions in a little while. If you are an elemental dieter you can take one of the instant-type breakfasts, or else eggs, meat, cheese, fish or peanut butter. And you should do this every morning. If you want to add some sweetening, you certainly can. As long as you take in a good supply of protein at the same time as the sugar, you're all right. The sugar will still cause a high level of insulin, but, since it's absorbed slowly, the protein will be available to keep the blood sugar up in the face of that increased insulin. It is when you take the sugar by itself in your sweet roll or pancakes that you are headed for sugar shock.

Sugar shock occurs when you eat a big breakfast of carbohydrates, such as pancakes (usually made from refined flour) covered with syrup. It is worse than no breakfast at all, and could even be harmful. The fellow or gal who goes off to work without breakfast can usually fire along toward lunch on the martinis, wine, baked meatballs and rutabagas from the night before. But remember the pancreas, our old overreacting friend, hiding there right behind the stomach? Well, a big breakfast of carbohydrates such as the pancakes and syrup feast makes this little devil absolutely blow his cool!

The massive ingestion of carbohydrates makes the pancreas fire off an enormous shot of insulin. The sugar hitting your bloodstream from the syrup and carbos in the pancakes makes the pancreas rev up as if it were preparing for a five-day orgy. As long as the pancakes are in the intestines and can sop up the insulin, you're okay. But the moment there is no further source of sugar, you're in sugar shock. The excess insulin drives the blood sugar into your cells, there is no longer any left for your brain and all types of bizarre symptoms suddenly appear.

Your stomach will ache with hunger cramps. Your head will swim and you will feel as if you were talking in a barrel. That funny, reverberating sound as though the ears are plugged is also a manifestation of excess insulin. As the symptoms progress, you will become confused, perhaps losing your comprehension of time and place, and irrational angers, fears and rages may come over you. Your vision will blur, you will have a headache, tension and a ringing in your ears.

Remember the last time you were frightened? Really scared or strung up with stage fright? Notice how similar these sugar shock symptoms are to fear symptoms. That is because low blood sugar and fear stimulate the same chemical, adrenalin. This is the basis of "uppers" that are sold illegally and keep one in a state of hyperaction. Low blood sugar kicks up the adrenalin because this is the chemical the body uses to raise the blood sugar. Once the adrenalin level is high enough, the blood sugar will raise to normal. But, oh, do you feel terrible!

Of course, since everybody is different, some of us do not suffer from low blood sugar under any circumstances. These people can wolf down a dozen glazed doughnuts and go on for hours. They are the lucky ones, so what we say here does not apply to them. Most people, however, will experience low blood sugar to a greater or less degree, even though only a few will have the disastrous symptoms described here. So if this description of sugar shock describes the way *you* feel, have your doctor check your blood sugar after a carbohydrate challenge. The glucose tolerance test should show up the problem, and making the diagnosis could even save your life.

So our big carbohydrate eater has taken on his refined-flour pancakes and syrup and a couple of hours later the hunger is getting him. If he has even the *tendency* to sugar shock he has only one choice at this point: he has to eat. If he is wise, he will use protein: nuts, cheese, even meat. If not, he will have to get the sugar in the form of a soft drink or candy bar to carry him through to lunch. But why go through that at all? It could be avoided easily just by starting the day with a big protein meal, something like those much maligned eggs we have talked about, or whole-grain breads, pancakes or waffles. Then there would be no problems with insulin sneaking up on you. The protein will be there in force till lunch time, pushing you along in good shape. There would be a pile of amino acids there too, to build whatever tissues your body needed through the morning. All those hundred trillion cells that have to be refurbished about every three weeks would have enough building blocks to form any number of tiny temples. Even on your way to work, or walking to the golf course, you can be rebuilding your body with fresh, new, vital, clean, healthy cells.

Exercise causes muscle destruction before it causes muscle rebuilding. The moment exercise is begun it demands an increase in the muscles' metabolic activity. The muscle cells wear out more quickly and must be discarded; new components must be manufactured at a faster rate. Actin and myosin molecules, blood vessels, cell walls, tough binding tissues that hold the muscle together, all of these must be built at a greatly increased rate. And all of these are formed from protein. No other food substance can be used to build any of these tissues anew.

Perhaps the best but least acknowledged reason for eating high protein for all three meals and whatever snacks you take is the fact that protein isn't habit-forming. That's right—it's not habit-forming. Carbohydrates are. That insulin mechanism we've been talking about makes it *extremely* habit-forming. The moment one reaches that low point in blood sugar, the moment sugar shock hits, one craves still more sugar. And the craving is bad. There is no habit like a chemical habit, and your body will scream for sugar to offset the insulin shots your pancreas is giving you. Not that namby-pamby fruit sugar, either. The body will crave the real thing, *refined* sugar! It tastes good, feels good and the inner man is comforted by it . . . for a little while. Maybe an hour or so. But the chain reaction has started to set in. With the new sugar, the pancreas secretes more insulin, and so on, until your typical carbohydrate eater becomes a chronic snacker. That's what that sweet tooth is all about. Look around at your friends—almost all of us know a chronic snacker, a sweet tooth who is hooked on carbohydrates and doesn't realize it. He cannot stand the feelings of sugar shock and continually is stuffing his face with more sugar in various forms to keep the blood sugar level up. He doesn't know enough, or is psychologically too weak, to break the whole disastrous action/reaction chain by ingesting high protein foods and forcing himself to give up sweets and high carbohydrate foods. No wonder obesity is epidemic in the land of refined sugar worshipers!

Protein simply will not cause the same effect. It doesn't fire off the insulin secretions and doesn't need the repeated feedings that carbohydrates need. It's an ideal diet food and a comfortable source of graded energy for the individual with an active physical life. For anyone starting my biotonic exercise program, protein is absolutely necessary—lots of it!

A sample diet could be as follows:

BREAKFAST:

Two eggs, any style, with bacon, ham or sausage, liver or chicken
Fruit juice
Wheat bread or rye toast, buttered
Milk or tea or coffee
Multiple vitamin

LUNCH:

Small steak, or liver
Lettuce salad with dressing
Whole wheat bread
Broccoli, cabbage or brussels sprouts
Coffee or tea
Fresh fruit of any kind or preserved fruit without sugar

DINNER:

Steak, roast, chops, chicken or fish—baked or broiled
Any two vegetables (beans, peas, corn, squash, etc.)
Baked potato
Fresh green salad
Fruit dessert

SNACK:

Natural cheese
Dry roasted nuts of any kind
One ounce cold meat (chicken, fish, sardines, oysters, clams, etc.)
Whole wheat crackers
Milk

One more plug for our friend, protein. It is a low volume food. Eating causes increased blood supply to the intestines. Any food, no matter how small a quantity, will bring this about. The larger the volume of food ingested, the greater the increased blood supply. Blood coursing through the intestines is then unavailable for supplying food to the delicate nipping of the brain. A lot of blood to the stomach is the most efficient means for digesting food, but not for thinking. That's why a large meal leads to that "post-prandial drag," the drowsiness that brings about the strong urge to take a nap, severely handicapping one's creative efforts. (Students, if you face a big morning exam, the breakfast outlined here will get you through. A snack of fruit or nuts just before the test might help further. But avoid all sweet foods that day. You can't afford sugar shock in the middle of the exam.)

In short, it takes a heap of pasta and potatoes to fill up the stomach, but a small steak or some tender liver or a couple of eggs can do the job nicely, and you'll never miss the volume.

That's my advice for all three meals, even for your late night TV snack. Our meal schedule in America right now is gravely unbalanced. Consider, we eat three full meals in eight hours, and we fast for sixteen. Does that make sense? For some it might work, but for a vast number of others it can't. The human body was not designed chemically and biophysically for that kind of nutritional imbalance. Are we, after all, at the mercy of the bus and train schedules? Is the world of commerce, the eight-hour shift, the nine-to-five daily routine, ruining our health by dictating this ridiculous eating schedule? Are the Latins right after all —doesn't a nice siesta after lunch, during the ten or twelve-hour work day, make more sense?

If you need a late night snack, snack on protein. Again, it's small in volume, burns slowly and satisfies the appetite.

And of course, it will make this exercise program work for you that much faster.

Here are the Five Commandments of Basic Nutrition:

First Commandment: It is not calories that make you fat. It is the *type* of food you eat.

Second Commandment: Carbohydrates are habit-forming, especially in the form of refined sugar. They may be delightful to eat, but they will be held accountable for your fat body. Wipe them out of your diet.

Third Commandment: Whole protein foods provide all the materials your body needs; in the proper proportions, they will not make you fat. Instead, they will build all the muscle, bone, enzymes, antibodies, hormones, cells and *sugar* you can possibly use.

Fourth Commandment: If you're exercising, the egg is your best friend. The mass media, having possibly endangered your health by sensationalizing the *only* bad effect of cholesterol, have neglected to tell you how *good* it is for you.

Fifth Commandment: Eat liver. Don't ask questions. I cannot remember any patients, men or women, having complained of fatigue or anemia if they liked, or regularly ate, liver. It is almost a perfect food, the best buy at your supermarket and extremely easy to prepare. If you "don't like" liver, acquire a taste for it. *Please!*

CHAPTER 6

Breathing: Harnessing an Ancient Power Source

Breathing is the universal burden. Every living organism on earth has some mechanism whereby it exchanges gases with its environment. Green plants pick up carbon dioxide and carbon monoxide and cycle these into plant food and energy, releasing oxygen. They began this perhaps a billion years ago, maybe more, and they converted the primitive atmosphere of methane and carbon dioxide into the one we know today, a mixture of nitrogen and oxygen. Roughly eighty percent nitrogen, an inert gas, and twenty percent oxygen, a very active gas.

Had animal life never developed, the primitive plants would have died. They would have fouled their nest with poisonous oxygen and passed out of the world. Even today there are many kinds of life that cannot live in an oxygen atmosphere.

Certain bacteria called anaerobes, for instance, are important in medicine and cause infections very difficult to treat.

But animal life obviously did develop to burn the oxygen back to carbon dioxide. Thus a balance has been struck between plants which use animal wastes as food and animals which use plant wastes.

But our interest is in human breathing and the mechanisms that go into it. Specifically, our interest is in using breathing power to improve posture and muscle tone.

I feel we should set this out quite clearly, for breath and its control have formed one of the powerful thrusts of some very profound philosophies—something we are not teaching.

Breathing is wired into the body in a uniquely important way. We must have two things: food energy and the oxygen to burn it. Food can be stored—in fact, some of us have stored so much we look like balloons. But oxygen cannot be stored. Therefore, we can live, at the very minimum, three or more weeks without food but only three minutes without oxygen. So we demand a minute-by-minute supply of oxygen and have developed a delicate system for its gathering.

Exactly why nature has not developed an oxygen storage system is unknown. Perhaps it is too difficult to store a gas, or maybe there has been such an abundance of oxygen for the past billion years it has never been found necessary. But we cannot store oxygen and the sixteen or so times a minute that we breathe are absolutely critical to life. However, studies show that we normally use only twenty percent of our lung capacity in regular breathing.

Many allusions have been made to our oxygen dependence. You need only see one man die by strangulation to be eternally impressed with its necessity; or to hold your own breath for a minute or so. In fact, right now, put down the book, take out your watch and hold your breath for a whole minute . . .

Tough, isn't it? You want to breathe so badly your lungs burst. You must use all your force to hold your mouth and nose closed. Your head swims, ears ring, vision darkens and horrible premonitions come upon you. These are all signs of carbon dioxide buildup in the blood and are all designed to force you to breathe. If you try to hold your breath until you die, you will simply pass out and automatically start breathing again. A powerful drive.

So we speak of the "breath of life" and equate breath with spirit. The lungs have been likened to the intellect and the yogis have grasped the breathing handle to forge a means of control over their entire being. They call this "controlling the prana" and have carried it to such a point as to bring breathing entirely under control of the mind. A marvelous feat, but what about the rest of us? We're not interested in such a high degree of control or such extreme discipline. We just want you to grasp the handle of *your* breathing enough, and only enough, to put this vital force to work on your muscles. If the yogi can grasp heaven with his breathing, you can grasp your gut muscles and learn to pull in your belly.

Stand in front of a mirror big enough to include your chest. You can see your ribs going from the flat place in front, your sternum, around to your back. Take a breath. Notice the ribs lift up and the spaces between them enlarge. These are the intercostal spaces and hold the intercostal muscles.

98

Take a big breath. Now the neck muscles bulge, the scalenus muscles and sternocleidomastoids stand taut and that big web of muscle from your neck to shoulders, the trapezius, stands out. As you face yourself, visualize your insides. The lungs fill their respective sides of the chest. Between them and right behind the sternum sits the heart. Feel for its beat and you will find it in the middle and over to your left. A strong heart thrust comes through about your left nipple. When you inhale and exhale you can see the extent of your lungs.

Now look at your neck. A deep inhalation pulls your Adam's Apple down, an exhalation pushes it up. The Adam's Apple, or larynx, is part of the trachea that moves air from the nose to the lungs.

Air comes in, preferably through the nose where it is warmed and filtered. It is drawn by the diaphragm and intercostal muscle actions down the trachea. At the bottom of the trachea the air goes two ways, into the right and left lung tubes or bronchi. Further branching of these bronchi leads to smaller and smaller tubes—called bronchioles—until the tiniest are reached, ending in the air sacs, or alveoli. Here the new air with its oxygen mixes with residual air in the air sac. The blood comes in very close contact with this air, gives up its burden of carbon dioxide and picks up oxygen.

A diagram of the blood system shows that all the blood in the body flows in a continuous circuit. Beginning at the left ventricle of the heart, blood goes out the systemic arteries, providing the cells of the body with oxygen and other nutrients. Passing through the capillaries, the blood is carried by the veins back to the heart—to the right auricle and the right ventricle. From there the blood passes into the pulmonary artery, where it is dark purple due to lack of oxygen. This artery brings the blood in contact with the lungs, so that it can give off the carbon dioxide it has collected and pick up fresh oxygen. It then passes to the pulmonary vein. By the time the blood has reached the pulmonary vein and drained into the left auricle it is bright red, full of oxygen and ready to go by way of the left ventricle back through the body.

The control mechanisms of this system are cybernetic miracles. It is a fallacy to believe the body does not need carbon dioxide. The body always maintains a proper level of carbon dioxide in the blood and in the alveoli and this chemical regulates the breathing and has an important role in allowing the body to handle acids and bases that otherwise would kill it. Carbon dioxide is measured in an area of the primitive brain so precisely as to always maintain exactly the proper level. The moment the blood level of carbon dioxide raises, respiration rate and depth increase so that carbon dioxide is discarded by the lungs. The moment blood carbon dioxide decreases, the rate and depth of respiration is decreased to hold carbon dioxide in the blood. The terrible efforts you were making to breathe a few minutes ago were triggered by an increase in carbon dioxide in the blood.

If you want to find out for yourself how vital carbon dioxide is to your well-being, start to breathe as fast and as deeply as you can; hyperventilate, as we say. Getting weak and dizzy? Notice your hands start to tingle? If you can keep this up long enough you will find your hands pulled into a kind of cone. The fingers are straight, bunched together, and the wrist is flexed. Notice, further, the moment you stop hyperventilating you no longer have to breathe. Several seconds will go by before your carbon dioxide builds up enough to again drive your respiration.

The hand tingling and subsequent position is an interesting study on what carbon dioxide does. This hand position is called a "carpopedal spasm" and is caused by a decrease in the available blood calcium. When one drives off the carbon dioxide with hyperventilation he makes the blood less acid. This allows some of the calcium to drop out of the blood, and there is insufficient calcium to relax the muscle and the carpopedal spasm results.

I'm sure every doctor remembers his first case of carpopedal spasm. The relatives rush a tense, white and rigid figure—perhaps a young lady—into the emergency room screaming, "Save her, doctor. She's having a seizure!" And the patient looks bad. Her face is taut, her arms and hands are pulled into a spasm and she's breathing like sixty. When the senior resident arrives he takes a paper sack, fits it tightly around her mouth and allows a few quiet minutes for the spasm to unlock and peace to reign. The sack served as a trap to catch the carbon dioxide the patient had been blowing off with her hysterical hyperventilation, allowing her blood carbon dioxide to build up to normal and making calcium available to her muscles.

One of the fallacies about breathing is that we should breathe deeply and "clean out our lungs." It certainly does no harm to breathe deeply; we ask you to do it in several of our exercises, but we do not ask you to hyperventilate. All this does is give you tingling hands.

"But you said you ordinarily use about twenty percent of your lung capacity. Shouldn't you exercise your lungs as you do your muscles?" This is a frequent question.

Exercise of the lungs is about as valuable as exercising a sponge. The lungs are big sacs full of alveoli with nothing to get stronger or better. Taking deep breaths slowly cannot hurt and may help to open a few extra alveoli. The exercises we ask you to do will exercise your lungs all you need. And you won't lose your lung reserve, unless you have an illness or subject your lung tissue to an irritant such as tobacco smoke.

"But my yoga instructor says I breathe incorrectly. I should breathe with my diaphragm instead of my chest."

Again, remember, yoga has different aims than we have. We are not teaching you to breathe, we are teaching you to use your breathing muscles to exercise themselves and other muscles. Singers learn to breathe with their diaphragms for very good reasons. If you learn diaphragm breathing and get a better feel of your belly muscles, great. Anything that increases such control is good.

Under ordinary conditions, however, until the lungs are hurt, diseased or overtaxed, we breathe precisely at the rate we need. Sitting calmly at our desk we breathe slowly and shallowly. Walking about the room both the rate and depth of respiration speed up. Running really pours on the coal and we open our mouths and drag in every bit of air we can. Even if our carbon dioxide drive mechanism should get out of whack we have a reserve system to back it up, the carotid body. This bit of tissue lying on the carotid artery in the neck is sensitive to arterial oxygen levels. If the oxygen drops, this body drives the respirations faster. Oxygen lack alone will keep you breathing.

Some diseases and toxic conditions interfere with the lung function. Breathing exercises should not be done until you have checked with your doctor.

Asthma is a crippling problem that can lower lung efficiency to very low levels. In this condition the lung traps air and its actual volume increases. But the tiny bronchioles that lead to the air sacs go into spasm and the flow of air is greatly slowed down. Smoking causes a similar condition in certain individuals, as we mentioned in Chapter 1, so both asthmatics and smokers will have a low air flow. This tends to increase their blood carbon dioxide on a continuing basis. The brain center that controls respiration resets itself at a higher level, so an even higher level of carbon dioxide is necessary to increase the respirations. Also, the smoker increases his carbon monoxide level and may have up to twenty percent of his hemoglobin tied up with carbon monoxide and not available to carry oxygen.

Both smoking and asthma lead to the medical horror called emphysema. This is a chronic overdistension of the lungs from the air trapping occurring in smokers and asthmatics. I remember the day *I* decided to quit smoking. Cancer has never frightened me because it is a reasonably fast death, but we had a whole ward full of patients with emphysema at the hospital where I trained. And these men had been pulmonary cripples for *years*. They were able to do little more than sit, bent forward, heads up, neck muscles working to get in enough air for life. They all had blue cheeks, pale lips and those odd, chubby fingers where the nail bends around the fingertip, called "clubbing."

The patient who really got to me was lying flat on his bed, arms over his head holding to the iron rods at the head of his bed. His arms were tense and he was pulling steadily. I walked in with three medical students.

"Why the position?" I asked, for it was the first time I had seen it.

"Doc, this is the only way I can breathe without fighting for air every minute."

I saw then that the arm position pulled his chest upward and gave him a little more room for air.

"Do you sleep that way?"

"As much as I ever sleep. Emphysema don't let you sleep much."

It was then I quit smoking.

Neither smokers nor asthmatics should do the breathing exercises. It is foolish to put further strain on lungs that are already hurt and these patients are more prone to pneumothorax than the nonsmokers and nonasthmatics.

Any pressure on the lungs can "blow out a bleb" in susceptible people. These blebs, like tiny blisters on the lung surface, are thin-walled sacs. When they rupture, air sneaks in between the chest wall and the lung and the lung collapses, a pneumothorax. You will know if this occurs as there is sudden pain and shortness of breath on the affected side. Patients with other less common lung ailments should consult their physician before beginning.

Let's go through two lessons in breathing now as a sort of warmup for the more formal exercises to come. These will help you understand something about the effect of the maneuvers and give you a little advance knowledge about them.

First, stand or sit erect, with your spine perfectly straight and your body relaxed. Then purposely protrude your belly as far out as you can, giving the diaphragm room to drop down and enlarge the chest activity. (This motion is like the "beer belly" effect we got when we were kids and wanted to make ourselves look fat.) At the same time you're pushing your stomach out, breathe in through the nose, drawing air into your lungs as deeply as you can. Imagine yourself filling your belly up with air, and continue to inhale until you feel your chest completely expanding, stretching, and you feel a tightness at the back of your throat. Soon you won't be able to inhale an iota more. Hold it for a moment and picture your blood circulating throughout the lungs and gobbling up all that fresh oxygen. Now, starting with the abdomen again, contract the stomach wall, pushing your diaphragm up against the bottom of the lungs. This action helps dispel the "dead air" that is usually sitting at the bottom of your lungs after each breath, but which is seldom expelled. Keep contracting your belly, forcing the air out. Do not take another breath until you can no longer contract your stomach and force more air out.

Now, as you are again holding your breath, notice that if you now suddenly protrude your stomach again, air will automatically be sucked into your lungs.

For our second demonstration, get a mirror and watch your face. Take a deep breath and tighten your belly muscles. If you do not know where these are, slip your hand between your belly and belt and push your hand against the belt by the force of your stomach muscles. Notice the minute you contract those muscles your face turns red, veins stand out on your neck like cords, your eyeballs bulge. If you look further over your body you will see all your hand and leg veins are full of blood.

Even a few moments, ten seconds, of hard straining against your belt makes you lightheaded and darkens your sight; these are the early signs of lack of oxygen to the brain. This happens because the straining pressure forces the blood to stay out in the veins, and keeps it away from the heart. That is why your veins swell up. Because the blood is not getting back to the heart, it is not available to supply the brain's needs. If you strain long enough, you will tumble over in a faint.

This taking a breath and straining with the belly muscles is an old exercise called the Valsalva Maneuver and has various medical applications. For instance, doing the Valsalva Maneuver while holding the nose will force air into the middle ear —a helpful act when you are coming down from a high altitude and your ears "plug up."

We encourage you to get familiar with Valsalva's old technique to learn the effects of breath control and be impressed by the profound changes such actions bring about throughout your whole body.

As you can see from all of this, we are almost teaching you to breathe all over again. To do our exercises, you need this extra instruction. The diaphragm and belly muscles are linked together. For the complete expansion of the lungs, the diaphragm must drop and the rib cage expand. This enlarges the chest cavity and enables the lungs to fill with good, fresh oxygen, like two balloons. It does this by extending the stomach wall, pushing the belly outward, thereby allowing the diaphragm to drop. This seesaw action of the two muscle groups, the belly and the diaphragm, is the basis of these breathing exercises.

You are using the most powerful method possible to harden the belly and chest muscles. Your lungs drive down on your belly like a pneumatic ram to fight with its muscles. Great muscle strength can be built quickly this way, but be very careful of the dangers mentioned under Valsalva's Maneuver.

CHAPTER 7

The Psychology of Exercise

What *really* drives someone to exercise? Why do people run, row, jump, climb, swim, play tennis? Why do people climb frozen mountains, risking their lives for what seems like nothing? Why do we pummel each other with leather gloves, jump out of airplanes, or glide on flimsy contraptions over canyons and cliffs? For money, glory, fame, adulation? Obviously. Or *is* it so obvious? When I watch a long distance runner practice hour after hour, legs aching, gut sick, lungs burning, I always wonder. Is it just money or glory that drives him? Really, it seems money could be easier to come by. Perhaps the superstars of organized sports do make enough money to pay for their pain, but what about the amateurs? The individuals jogging a mile each night, playing handball in the afternoon, giving up lunch to swim—these people are not in it for money or glory or anything but the brief fun of playing with their friends or a painful workout alone.

I would like to kick these questions around with you before you tackle your exercise. Maybe in finding your own answers, far better ones than I can give, you will strike the well of your motivation and get carried through your twelve weeks. After that you should be hooked enough to work out at least once a week.

It has been shown in laboratory experiments that rats deprived of their whiskers died within a short time, primarily because they were unable to comprehend their environment. The rats were too "worried" and "apprehensive" because, as with most animals, having lost their primary means of exploration, in this case their whiskers, they were unable to find out about their environment.

Many of us are like that. We act as though we had lost our ability to sense our environment and we fall back on our derrieres and refuse even to explore the possibility of becoming fit and the advantages it might offer. We know we should, but we put it off and put it off, and then it is too late. Our muscles are too frail to stand the strain, bones too brittle and joints far too arthritic to put up with such activity. But we know we should do it and we worry and stew about it and compound our problem. We add the pain and energy drain of worry to the flabby, depleted body. No wonder we become tired, sluggish, overweight and mentally slow.

Any doctor knows what I mean here. His office is full of such patients. They are a weary lot. Any layman knows at least a hundred such. They are the sad and mopey ones, always tired. They sleep poorly, badger their physician for sleeping pills which leave them hung over the next morning and have a terrible time getting going. All day they are tired, their feet hurt, backs ache, bellies hurt, and life is a mountain of misery and hopelessness. They trudge into the office like lost souls. One wonders if Dante had an office full of such patients when he wrote his *Inferno*.

We run test after test on blood, urine and tissues and we X-ray and probe and search and we find nothing. There is no organic basis for the problem; these patients are victims of their own worry. Worry is an ice blue fear that steals over warm, pink faces and pulls on vibrant bodies, draining the life out of them like a terrible succubus. I appeal to these people and attempt to reach into their fears with rational words, but usually it is of no help. Women trapped in loveless marriages, men dreading to go home to the constant nagging of their coldly critical wives, people frustrated with their position in life—all these souls begging for recognition.

There are four human needs and we have addressed two of them. They are food, oxygen, water and recognition. Water needs little discussion. You drink enough not to be thirsty and that's about it. But recognition is the problem of everyone in every society at every time. We want to be recognized "for ourselves." The most beautiful girl on the block bemoans the fact she is just a sex object and the most handsome man worries because he isn't listened to at the Chamber of Commerce meeting. Talented musicians, athletes, scholars, artisans, artists, are all the same. They all want to be recognized "for themselves." Our teen-agers wear their hair long, their Levi pants patched and torn and their shirts hung out but that is all right because what really matters is what's inside.

This is the crux of it. If we can be recognized for what we are, for ourselves, for "the real me," there would be a lot less sad, weary, tired, hung over, aching people on the earth and the doctors' offices would be less full.

Can these exercises help this problem? Yes, indeed they can. Listen as we review the logic that lead to this conclusion.

What is it that we actually recognize in our friends, family and acquaintances? Immediately you think of income, social position, physical prowess, and these are all correct. But there is one common denominator to all these, one word that slips under them all and can be traded for them. That word is "discipline." And the best discipline is *self*-discipline.

There is no question such discipline is universally admired. What is more galling than working with a promiser who is always telling you he will do such-and-such but who never has the discipline to deliver? Is a maiden's dream a man with a belly hanging over a sagging belt who hasn't the discipline to train it and lose weight? After the last baby, was the twenty pounds you gained "glandular" or just lack of discipline? Why isn't your body firm and your mind alert? Because you lack discipline?

Well, stand up and be counted. Get back in the mainstream and out of the tide pools of life. Here are the elements of exercise and diet to firm, thin and shape you back to an attractive soul and do it so secretly even your spouse need not know.

Food, health and physical fitness go hand in hand, and the psychological message is clear: to feel healthy, you must be fit. Many people think health is merely the absence of disease. This could not be further from the truth. If a person is always listless, hates to get out of bed, and so on, he isn't healthy.

Winston Churchill said, "The man who works with his muscles all day, should work with his mind at night. The man who works with his mind all day, should work with his muscles at night." And old Winston was right. A sound mind does indeed go with a sound body, and vice versa.

In his book, *Yoga Made Easy,* Desmond Dunne tells the story of a UNESCO team of health experts visiting the Balkans shortly after World War II. During the visit, a doctor interested in mother-child problems happened upon a group of peasant women in a remote Bulgarian village. Chatting with them, she noticed a beautiful young woman whom she guessed to be about twenty-five, and who turned out to be the wife of a local dignitary. The dignitary, a huge, virile type, was well into his nineties. Having buried his fourth wife, he apparently had suggested marriage to this lusty girl, who had been flattered and accepted him. Nine months after their marriage, a child was born.

The incredulous UNESCO doctor made some inquiries. She tried to get the young wife to tell about the tribe's sexual customs. Perhaps, she hinted, there was some socially acceptable ritual of stand-ins, or surrogate sex partners, in the instance of such May-December pairings. When the girl seemed puzzled, obviously having no idea what the UNESCO doctor was hinting at, the doctor became more direct: did her elderly spouse really still enjoy sex? The young mother was wide-eyed with surprise. Of course! Was the doctor trying to say that it was otherwise in that part of the world where *she* came from?

The lesson of the old man and the young bride is important, not only for the sexual implications, but also for the whole idea of *attitude*. The old man didn't *know* he was supposed to become impotent and senile with age, as we westerners seem to insist on. He simply kept doing what came naturally.

It's the same with exercise and physical fitness. If we get ourselves "psyched up" for getting into physical shape, we'll not only exercise better, we'll feel better for doing it. This, in turn, will have a self-propelling effect. The better we feel, the more we'll exercise. It isn't much different psychologically from quitting smoking, wherein the first day off cigarettes gives us the strength to try harder to make it through the second day.

Being fit doesn't mean we're ready to enter the decathalon, either. Americans seem to believe there are only two kinds of people—athletes and spectators. Further, they believe that only the athletes need to "stay in shape." This is totally wrong. Everyone needs to stay in shape, and everyone can accomplish it, to one degree or another. But it starts with your state of mind, your attitude.

Getting into shape usually is a yearly ritual that starts shortly after New Year's Day and lasts for about two weeks. The eager resolver gets up early and jogs for a while, usually with a friend who has also made the resolution to "get in shape." (This is usually accompanied by "going on the wagon" for a while, too.) After the jogging novelty wears off (or during it), the exercise enthusiast plays tennis more often, or starts swimming a few laps every day. Maybe he or she will walk or bicycle to work

113

a few times, or park further away than usual to walk a longer distance to the office. Maybe he or she will take the stairs instead of the elevator, do some light weightlifting, start dancing classes or take up some other regimen. All well and good.

However, in the evening after work he'll celebrate his new program with a few drinks and a big dinner. He'll turn in early and sleep the sleep of babes, because he's exhausted. In the morning he'll awake with aching muscles, discover that further exercise is painful, probably decide to lay off until the muscles "loosen up" and finally come to the conclusion that exercise is for younger people.

Think about your biotonic program. As you read these pages, begin to think about getting into shape, about becoming stronger, achieving more endurance and vitality. I know many people who weren't able to give up smoking or drinking until they had thought about it for a while, psyching themselves up, conditioning their *spirits* to accept a new way of life. Start slowly. Think some more. Do just a few exercises, and *think* about what you've done. Lord knows, we've got plenty of time to think during the standard day. Start thinking about your body. Start being *vain!* Look in the mirror often and imagine your body as you want it to look. Think about it when you are eating, as well as when you are exercising. During an exercise, think about what's happening to you. In the description of each exercise I've included a brief analysis of what's actually happening to your muscles and body. *Think* about that as you perform each one.

Exercise is boring, most of the time. Thinking about what you're doing helps overcome this. Remind yourself of your goals, and measure your progress often. Be realistic. Don't try to accomplish too much in too short a time. Remember, it took your body a certain length of time to become soft and fat and weak—give yourself some time to change all that.

And think good thoughts. Think sex thoughts. Exercise certainly can alter your sex life as it changes the rest of your life. Obviously, you will look better. You will lose a few pounds, pull in your gut, lift up your head to see what's happening in the world about you. Your physical appearance tightens, strengthens and improves. Like the athlete.

He has a firm body with powerful muscles, quick reflexes and beautiful tone. His carriage is lithe and erect and a healthy glow burns at his cheek. We are talking about the competitive athlete, the basketball, swimming or tennis challenger who exerts his whole body and expends his energy on the playing field.

But dare we believe the whispered reports? Is this superbeing less than the world's greatest lover? Well, maybe he is. During times of exertion the male athlete, at least, becomes less than an ideal sex object, because it has been shown that the male body runs out of testosterone before its other hormones are exhausted. Long distance runners, when studied, still had plenty of cortisone and other necessary body components, but their testosterone fell. This hormone testosterone puts the lover into love. Without it a male cannot have any sex desire. It is the hormone that is produced at puberty, brings about the male sex characteristics and directs the sex life. Much testosterone equals much sex and little testosterone equals little sex.

So, the male athlete will have no sex interest immediately after the contest until his testosterone rebuilds.

Mentally, too, athletes have to put other goals before sex. Long, grueling and painful training sessions are daily fare. A terrible tenacity toward physical perfection must drive them like obsessed demons. On the field there can be only one victor and the challenger willing to give that extra time and suck in that extra pain will be the victor. Such an athlete may not really have enough time or enough energy for sex. Nor enough of the tender, yielding, gentle emotions that make sex a rapture instead of a rape.

But the out-and-out sexist is looking for a compromise, the body of an athlete with the energy and lusts of a satyr. And satyrs were notorious for lying around and being indulged by nymphs. In an oblique way, and in a rather sneaky fashion, the biotonic exercises outlined in this book might just accomplish this, for these are compromise exercises.

A beautiful body? Fine carriage? Strong bones? Indeed, range of motion and biotonic exercises can accomplish this. All the joints are kept supple, the muscles are built into smooth, bulging curves and the posture made perfect. The back strengthening exercises are designed for posture, encouraging the flat belly, straight back, balanced gait of the athlete. And these exercises are based on the very basic motion of sex itself, the pelvic tilt. All the muscles that thrust the pubis upward in the pelvic tilt, thrust it forward in sex. All these exercises develop stamina and staying power and encourage extended performance.

Also, these exercises do not deplete the male or female hormones relating to sex. They do not deplete anything. They build only. America may be looking to a renaissance of sex.

Psych yourself up—you're ready to go!

PART TWO

The 12-Week Biotonic Program for Strength and Stamina

CHAPTER 8

The Range of Motion Exercises

This first group of exercises is designed to increase the range of motion (ROM) of your joints. That is their only function. These are the most universally applicable exercises for protecting and improving joint function. The only time one could *not* do these would be in the throes of acute rheumatoid arthritis. But, even then, putting the inflamed joint through as much motion as possible without causing undue pain might be a good idea. This is an area that *must* be checked with one's own physician before anything is done. Except for that disease, however, I believe anyone can do these exercises anywhere, to great advantage.

These exercises make good sense. They are the ideal introduction to the more strenuous, complicated—and sometimes painful—exercises to follow in the section on strength and stamina. By themselves they can alleviate a lot of joint problems and make you a more fluid, supple person. They can avoid muscle pulls, strains and sprains. Surgeons have their offices full of joint-related problems, and many of these would never have arisen with proper ROM exercise programs. We see innumerable patients coming in with their arms pinned to their sides and that desperate look on their faces, clutching the affected area—mostly the shoulder—for dear life. They have the deeply etched look of pain after having stayed up nights pacing the floor with bursitis or tendonitis. More poor souls than I care to remember come in with their knee joints ground away and swollen from being too fat and from doing nothing to strengthen the muscles around those joints. Many of our part-time athletes, living out the dreams of high school, some of them close friends of mine, are out on the handball or squash court pounding the lining out of their joints and refusing to do even the simple ROMs we will detail here. They crave the glory of competition and totally ignore the protection of their joints.

The thrill of victory, the agony of defeat—remember? Let's change that to "the thrill of physical health, the agony of smashed or stiffened joints." Now that skiing has become a national rage we are going to have to keep in some kind of shape when the snow is *off* the ground. One cannot go to the slopes at the first snow, after only a few knee bends and push-ups, and expect not to get hurt. You can't take joints that aren't properly mobile and throw them against the kind of stress one gets in skiing and expect to escape unscathed. Even though you might not *feel* it, you are damaging your joints when you fail to exercise them properly before any physical exercise. These ROMs will help immeasurably, and the strength and stamina exercises that follow will do wonders for your performance.

America is a land that refuses to grow old. We want to stay young and vital into old age, and we don't even want to call it "old age." So we must get that old woman's hump out of our backs and that old man's droop out of our shoulders. We must keep the joints supple and moving. We must get up and *do* something!

Even the most compulsively active of us have to have some kind of goal, some means of measuring where we are and whether we're making progress. The tennis players can go up their ladders from C to B to A; the golfers have their score cards; the runners their times and distances; the weight-lifters their weights; the skiers their slopes and the sky-divers their heights and targets. I promised you no fancy equipment or required clothes, and I meant it, so I've devised a few ways to measure your progress at home, at your leisure. If you have a bathroom scale, place it under a door jamb and stand on it, pushing upward as hard as you can. You can look down and see how far you can move the dial, and record this. Do it every week, to see whether it's increasing. Another way is to do push-ups, that time-honored calisthenic where you lie on the floor face down and, body stiffened, push up with your hands and arms as many times as you can. Or if you have a friend who's a physical therapist, he could measure your strength, or if you really want, you could invest in a small set of weights for very little money and do some weight-lifting along with my recommended exercises. I'm counting on your becoming so impressed with your progress, that you'll want to continue some kind of strenuous regimen for some time. My comments on weight-lifting will help you here. Most people understand weight-lifting only in the "body beautiful" sense—not as exercise. But weight-lifting is very good exercise. It is slow, yet vigorous, strenuous, and one is seldom injured by it. It can serve as an ideal accompaniment to our biotonics, and works well for warm-up kinds of exercising. And unless you actually make a dedicated, obsessive *attempt* to look like Arnold Schwartznegger, you won't!

Okay, here we go. ROMs may be done at any time during the day, and during almost any activity. I'll indicate when might be a good time to do each, so that you may be "reminded" to do them at various times of your daily schedule. Many of us perform certain functions regularly, such as showering, brushing teeth, going to and from work, shopping, cleaning, reading, driving and so on. Even in the bathroom, we can perform certain ROM exercises without surrendering any of our precious time. Remember always that wherever and whoever you are, you can stretch almost anytime you wish. And you can contract anytime you wish, too.

Exercise 1

The Clutch

Open the hand wide, separating the fingers, palms up. Really stretch it out. Now curl the fingers slowly inward, trying to begin at the joints at the tips, and rolling them slowly into the palm to create a tight fist, as if you are slowly clutching an object and trying to crush it.

This exercise puts in motion all the small muscles of the hand, more than a dozen of them whose names are too esoteric to delineate here. It also puts a good stretch on the muscles originating in the forearm which curl or flex the fingers, together with those which extend the fingers. This makes the joints firm and supple, and assures adequate motion. Instead of the hollow spaces that lie between your fingers, you will notice even bulges which are smooth and rounded. Women will develop more beautiful fingers and be proud to show off nail polish and rings, for smooth and attractive fingers are a mark of beauty.

Fingers can easily become damaged from various causes, including arthritis, and careful stretching such as this can keep them supple. This stretching may even be painful. But I believe that at least some of the crippling that goes along with arthritis could have been avoided by early application of finger exercises.

"The Flower" is a variation of this exercise. Instead of curling all the fingers inward at once, do them one at a time, beginning with the pinky. Note how all the other fingers follow in turn, as if a delicate flower is folding up for the night, then opening up again with the morning sunshine.

Do these five times only for each hand. Good times to do them are while driving a car, or simply while walking down the street. They are easily camouflaged in public.

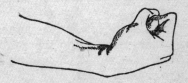

The Wrist Twist

With the hand relaxed, palm down, bend the wrist as far backward as it will go, then as far forward. Now do it from right to left. In each case, go as far as the joint will allow, and then try for a bit further. Here you are stretching the small muscles of the hand, the interossei and lumbricales, the large flexors lying in the forearm on what is called the volar surface (the palm side) and the extensors lying on what is called the dorsal surface (the back of the hand side).

This exercise gives you a strong wrist, with some forearm byproduct benefits. As the wrist's strength and flexibility is mandatory for many sports and work activities, this should be done as often as you can, perhaps in many situations when you are sitting, such as waiting in an office, while reading (do it with the hand that isn't holding the book) or after dinner. Naturally, you would also benefit

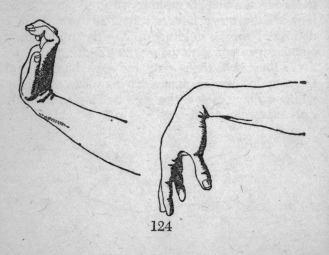

124

from doing this before your tennis game. Remember that the force of the entire arm goes through the wrists, and a freely pivoting joint is useful in almost every sport.

The Fist Wrist Twist

Again with palms down, make a fist and perform the same movement as the Wrist Twist, except this time *roll* your wrist through a 360-degree roll. At every point in the roll the fist should be as fully bent as possible. Now reverse the motion and roll the other way.

Clenching the fist adds a powerful strain on the flexor muscles of the forearm. If you wrap your free hand around your forearm as you begin this exercise, you'll feel the muscle tense. Eventually it will become hard as a rock. Just clenching the fist brings about a whole new balance of muscles as you'll see when you've done them for a few days, and you can feel where it hurts. With the muscles of the wrist very tightly clenched, one begins to bring into play all the force of static thrust and the enormous strengthening that goes with it.

As with the finger exercises, the exercises for the wrists can be done virtually anywhere, and are easily camouflaged in public. Do them as often as

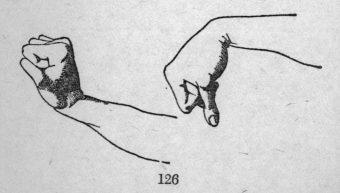

you want. (An especially good time to do these is while you are getting chewed out by the boss—your fists are clenched anyway, why pass up the opportunity?)

Elbow Bend #1

Standing erect, hands at side, bend your elbow by bringing your hand, palm upward, toward the shoulder as far as it will go. Stretch hard on this one. Try to grasp your shoulder with your hand, but leaving the hand relaxed. Now straighten your elbow again and let your hand come to rest at your side.

The biceps and triceps are the two muscles that are most powerfully affected here. But the forearm and shoulder muscles are also stretched. The biceps are the lifting muscles; triceps are throwing, punching, pushing muscles.

Remember how important this joint is by considering it for a moment. You couldn't feed yourself if it were not for the elbow, nor comb your hair, wash your face, shave, blow your nose . . .

This exercise lubricates this important joint and keeps the bursa sacs healthy and secreting their critical juices. Fractures of the elbow frequently result in loss of extension of this joint, necessitating strong exercise efforts to get the joint aligned again.

Do these five times each, alternating arms. For

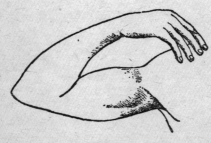

most people, combing the hair would be an excellent time to perform these, since you are essentially doing the motion anyway. Or when zipping up the back of your dress, knotting your tie or shaving.

Elbow Bend #2

Make a tight fist this time and bend the elbow as in Elbow Bend # 1. The tighter the fist, the better the muscle tension. Bring it as close to your shoulder as you can. Notice how the elbow still moves as easily, but that this time you are putting additional strain on the forearm and bicep.

Do five times for each arm.

This is another exercise designed to gradually introduce you to static thrust maneuvers (to follow). The tight fist throws a strain on the hand and forearm muscles, but it also tenses the muscles acting across the elbow joint; thus, the biceps and triceps must work much harder to alternately bend and extend the elbow. In turn, the shoulder muscles are more tense. The benefit from this is obvious—greater tension of these muscles sets all the arm joints more perfectly in their respective sockets and puts strengthening stress on the muscles.

Any time you wish to show off your biceps muscle is a good time to do this one, such as on the beach, in the shower or, hopefully, in the bedroom.

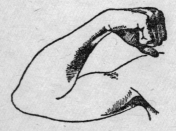

The Tennis Non-Elbow

(This exercise is also called "the Mezzo-Mezzo," in honor of an Italian friend's gesture for "so-so.")

Stand erect, arms at sides. Bend the elbow at a right angle bringing your palm face up, as if receiving some money. Next rotate your palm inward until it is face down. Continue to rotate it as far as you can without bringing your elbow out from your side. Now reverse the movement and rotate your palm back to face up position, continuing as far as you can in that direction. Feel the tension in your upper forearm and elbow.

In this exercise you are using a set of muscles not ordinarily exercised: the pronator and the supinator, lying around the elbow joint and acting to "pronate" (turn down) and "supinate" (turn up) the hand.

This exercise and the one to follow bring the remarkable rotational ability of the elbow and forearm into play. It is a very delicate mechanism, depending on the ligaments around the elbow joint for its performance. Tennis elbow, a very painful

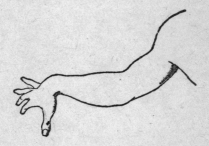

and common condition involving inflammation of the rotator cuff surrounding the head of the radius bone, may be prevented by this exercise. I had the condition myself and performed this exercise quite religiously and it went away. Anyone playing competitive tennis or any other sport which puts undue strain on the elbow should do this exercise on a regular basis. And while you may always serve (which usually brings tendonitis of the elbow) with the same arm, don't forget to do this exercise for *both* arms!

You can do this only once or twice a day for the first week, then increase it to five times or more, as comfort permits.

The Fonz

This is essentially the same as the Tennis Non-Elbow, except for balling your hand into a tight fist when performing it. Now the exercise becomes a powerful exerciser of the rotator muscles to the elbow, working against the resistance of the forearm muscles. It tightens the rotator cuff around the radius bone as well.

Do this once or twice a day, until comfort permits more. However, before starting to do the Fonz regularly, do the Tennis Non-Elbow (or the Mezzo-Mezzo) at least for a full week. The Fonz throws the force of forearm contractions across the pronators and supinators and puts a much greater strain against them. Therefore, this is more effective than the Tennis Non-Elbow and much more strenuous. Whenever one feels in the mood for a gesture of derision, we recommend the Fonz. If you don't feel derisive, do it when you are driving your car.

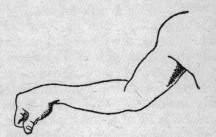

ROM SHOULDER EXERCISES

The exercises I have developed for the shoulder are perhaps the most important ROM exercises I can share with you. I would bet that almost every reader knows *someone* who has either shoulder or back problems. Shoulder problems occur as we grow older because we haven't been exercising our shoulder joints while we were jogging, dieting, golfing or whatever. The shoulder tends to be ignored, simply because as long as we can *move* it, we think it's fine. The fact of the matter is that your shoulder tightens up without your even knowing it until the movement suddenly becomes so restricted that you start feeling pain. Shoulder joint problems can be a lot like drinking vodka—you don't know you've gone too far until it's too late!

I have but to think of my last patient with shoulder problems. A fine, strong man, a rancher, who had the North Dakota disease of tendonitis. (This is quite common in this region, although no one seems to know why. Elsewhere, they have bursitis, but here we experience much more tendonitis of the long tendon of the biceps muscle.) My patient came in as they all do, holding his shoulder with his good hand, cuddling it close to his body. Even his usually stoic face showed the agony and lack of sleep he'd been through already. It had degenerated to the point of the shoulder becoming completely frozen, i.e., having no motion in the joint whatsoever. I had to hospitalize him, put him to sleep, inject cortisone into the joint and manipulate it while he was out.

There is no more sickening sound—or feel—in the world than the crunchy, grinding *snap!* a frozen joint makes when it finally breaks loose. It sounds like it has broken forever and will never move again. I have seen seasoned nurses turn pale when they hear it. But the man now has a free joint with no pain. He shouldn't have had it frozen in the first place, but no one had told him the importance, even in his occupation as a hard-working rancher, to exercise that crucial joint and keep it moving.

Tendonitis, whatever its cause, runs the same course. Always there is the aching pain in the shoulder; the patient attempts to relieve this by holding the shoulder close to his body, adhesions set up in the shoulder joint that glue it down tight, the pain worsens, he cuddles it more and in this vicious cycle the joint freezes solid. By the time the patient gets to this point nothing but surgical manipulation will help. *But,* if active ROM and S&S exercises are begun early, full ROM can be maintained and the condition controlled.

Another case comes to mind. A young man, quite strong, who had already been diagnosed as having rheumatoid arthritis, came to me with almost completely frozen shoulders. His physician believed in the "rest" theory of arthritis treatment, and had decided to immobilize his patient's shoulders for this reason. In this particular case, it had led to almost frozen shoulders. We agreed that he would try to move them, to exercise them, even if it hurt like hell. For him, we chose a set of weights and got him exercising regularly on ROMs. It was amazing. Within a very brief time one couldn't tell he'd had arthritis at all, and now when I see him regularly he is free from pain and has complete motion of all joints, even though his extremities are still unusually warm (a symptom of arthritis).

Please understand, now, that I don't advocate exercising for all types of arthritis, nor do I feel it will always help. All the exercises do is maintain the ROM of the joint while the disease is quieting down. If you think you have arthritis, go to your doctor and have the tests run. That is mandatory.

I have tendonitis in my own shoulders and have to keep them exercised. As long as I exercise them regularly, I have no pain. But let me slack off on my exercises for a while, and I experience the dull, aching pain again. So I have personal experience to buoy my faith in these exercises.

Exercise 8

Let Your Fingers Do the Walking

Reach up and touch the back of your neck with your first two fingers. Now let your fingers do the walking . . . down your spine. Creep downward a bit and feel a bony prominence, which is the spine knob at the base of your neck, the spinous process of the seventh neck vertebra. Now, start "walking" your fingers down your spine, touching each spinous process as if your fingers were jumping from rock to rock across a stream: Walk them as far down as you can, reaching a little further each time you go.

In the process of walking down your spine, you are putting a powerful strain on the joint capsule of the shoulder. This structure is designed to limit the up-and-back motion of the shoulder, the earliest motion to be lost when the shoulder becomes stiff. Therefore, you are continually gaining that last little bit of motion that keeps your shoulder pain-free. (You are also exercising the deltoid muscle, all the muscles around the shoulder blade, and that great climbing muscle, the latissimus dorsi.) Lifting the arm higher than the head becomes a colossal accomplishment when you start having arthritic problems of the shoulder.

An excellent time to do this exercise, ladies, is when you are reaching down your back for your zipper. I hope our men have enough back itches to remind them of this exercise.

Do this exercise five times with each arm.

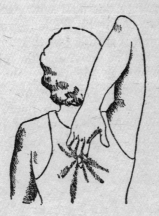

The Back Scratcher

Reach around your back at the belt line until you're touching your spine. Now move the hand, with the thumb leading the way, as far *up* the spine as it will go. This is essentially the reverse of the previous exercise. Stretch further each time you do it. These exercises were shown to me by an excellent orthopedist who assured me that these alone would keep the shoulders free and mobile, and I have become a disciple.

Don't forget to do these with each arm. As in Let Your Fingers Do the Walking, you are stretching the shoulder capsule, but this time in a different direction. The combination of these two exercises should, as my orthopedic friend says, give you complete shoulder motion.

The muscles involved in the Back Scratcher are primarily the biceps, the muscles to the thumb and those that pull the shoulder tightly to the body,

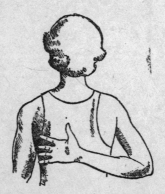

such as the rhomboideus major and minor, and the serratus anterior.

Anytime is a good time for this exercise. Leaning against the wall at a cocktail party, waiting at a train station or when looking at the moon.

The Confidence Strut

When you've done the previous exercises for about three weeks, you should then be able to join hands behind your back with one arm reaching down your spine and the other reaching up.

With the fingers linked together (or hands grasped, if you're *really* limber!), strut around the room on your toes. Get the feeling of confidence, of self-accomplishment, of *power*. None of your friends, I'll bet, will be able to do this, and they'll become alarmed at the rigidity of their shoulder joints. Lord it over them. After all, what do *they* know?

Change hands and do it again. Do the Confidence Strut whenever you feel like it, especially

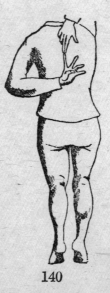

when depressed. It's a good one for late in the day, when changing clothes after work or before dinner, or anytime you feel sad, blue, paranoid, put upon or abused. Or anytime you want to cheer up someone *else* in the room, since no one can watch this exercise being done without smiling.

The Softball Pitch

Stand erect. Hold the arm straight out from the body, to the side, keeping the wrists and elbow straight. Now begin a slow circular movement, as if you were standing beside a blackboard and trying to draw a circle on it. Gradually make the circle larger and larger until you are swinging your arm in a vertical plane, much like a softball pitcher's delivery.

Now reverse the direction of the circle, and then do it with your other arm. Do each until you start feeling foolish.

In this exercise, you are actively stretching the

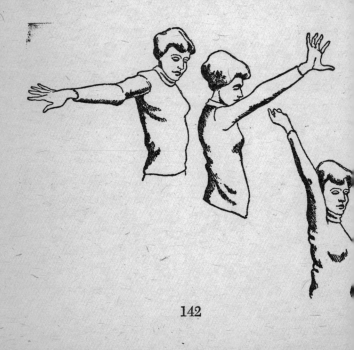

shoulder capsule in both directions. But don't be fooled—you cannot get the stretch that you can in Exercises 8 and 9, so do *not* substitute the Softball Pitch for 8 or 9. Also, you are not exercising your shoulder muscles very much with the Softball Pitch, so use this exercise only to warm up and get ready for the tougher ones.

Reach for the Sky!

Stand erect and put your arms straight above your head. Now reach back as far as you can . . .

Bend your elbows as far as they'll go, then straighten your arms out fully. Really get up on your toes and reach back as hard and as far as you can.

Done properly, this will provide shoulder stretching equivalent to Let Your Fingers Do the Walking. The deltoids, teres major and minor, and the trapezius muscles are strained. Anytime you feel like stretching is an excellent time for this exercise. I know of no better relief for an aching shoulder bombarded with tendonitis or bursitis than this exercise. It can be done anywhere and has the nice side-effect of loosening the back of the neck.

Do at least five of these and, for comfort's sake, even ten.

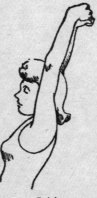

The Anita Ekberg Kroner Holder

Stand erect and hold out your arms in front of you, fingers touching. Now swing the arms out to the sides as far as they'll go back, until you feel your shoulder blades squeezing together. Try to touch your shoulder blades together, pretending you can hold a coin between them. Now bring the arms back in front and relax. Do this again five times.

As the shoulders swing backward, the rhomboids and serratus muscles are powerfully strained, and the rhomboids particularly tensed to pull the shoulder blades together. Strengthening these muscles and moving the shoulder joints is good conditioning for digging in the garden, cleaning the garage and attic, and chopping firewood. The exercise is so named because it will give you a broad, strong and shapely back. If just the second portion, pulling the shoulders together, is done, the exercise may be done anywhere and completely without anyone's knowledge. Do this every time you feel like stretching or scratching.

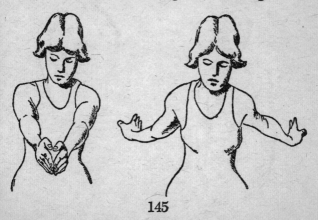

Jack the Clapper

The name of this exercise comes from a combination of an Overhead Clap and the standard Jumping Jack. It's simple. Start with your arms at your sides and simply swing them up and clap your palms together above your head, then bring them back to your sides. The important thing in this exercise is to stretch your arms outward *as far as they'll go* while bringing your hands overhead.

A variation of this is the classic calisthenic Jumping Jack, where you jump, spreading your legs, at the same time you clap your hands overhead.

I've included this rather prosaic exercise because it provides quick ROM work for almost all the joints of the body and vast comic relief for my more corpulent readers. If you can't do any of the other exercises, if you forget them, if you never itch, scratch or stretch, you can still steal off in

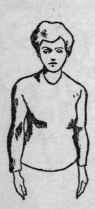
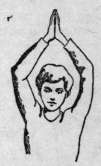

the quiet of your own bedroom, in front of your full-length mirror and clap yourself up and down ten times. Repetitive use of this exercise will provide all the benefits of jogging or a quiet tennis game. Apartment dwellers, finding themselves confined, can avail themselves of this quick and easy overall conditioner. Be merciful on the people downstairs.

Do this exercise as many times as you care to, until you find yourself out of breath. Count how many you can do, and start trying to better your record every time.

The Bending Butterfly

We seldom perform any maneuvers with our hands behind our backs, and this has a restrictive effect on the back motion of the shoulder joint. Stretch your hands in front of you, backs of the hands together, as if beginning a butterfly stroke. Now stretch your arms outward as far as they can go, while slowly *doing* that butterfly, until you can clasp your hands behind your back, arms still outstretched.

Now, keeping your hands clasped, bend forward slowly while forcing your clasped hands upward as high as they'll go. Eventually your head should be around your knees, and your hands where your head was when you were standing erect.

This gives an unusual looseness to the shoulders in a direction which will lubricate the entire joint. This is actually a combination exercise, given in

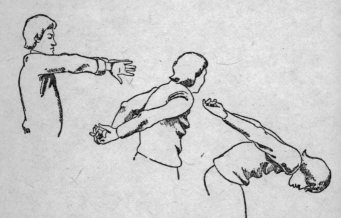

case, due to laziness or time pressures, you've been eliminating any of the other shoulder exercises.

Do it five times.

Neck-and-Neck

I know an orthopedic surgeon who knocks over his garbage cans and anything else in his driveway every time he backs his car out, simply because his neck is so stiff he can't look over his shoulder to see behind him. I mention him to emphasize the importance of the neck joint, and often we need the use of it even in the most mundane of daily motions.

This is a double exercise. First, rotate the neck and head so that you are trying to look behind you. Turn all the way to the right and see how far behind you can see. Then turn to the left and do the same. Stretch your head around as far as you can in each direction.

Second, let your head fall onto your right shoulder as far as it will go. Try to touch your ear to your shoulder. Reverse it and do the same with the left shoulder.

During each of these you may hear a cracking, grating sound in your neck. These are calcium deposits, and they are breaking up as you perform these motions. If allowed to build up sufficiently,

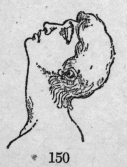

your head would become totally immobile and wouldn't even be able to nod "yes" or "no."

Do five of these each, but do them as often as you like during your daily routine.

The Neck Roll

Start with your chin on your chest, trying to touch it as tightly as you can. Then, rotate your head back over your right shoulder, keeping the neck stretched to the side as far as it will go, and proceed all the way until you are looking up at the ceiling as your head moves to the back. Now, being sure your head is back *as far as it will go,* continue the rotation until you are coming back across your left shoulder and finally wind up with your chin on your chest again. I will wager that during the first time you do this exercise you will feel the calcium deposits crunching in your joints. Reverse the motion and rotate your head the other way.

There is no reason you cannot do this exercise every day of your life from now on, at least five rotations a day in each direction.

This is especially designed to strengthen the sternocleidomastoid muscles. These are the bands that stand out on the neck when it is turned to either side. Both will act to prevent that forward, old age look when the head hangs slouched in

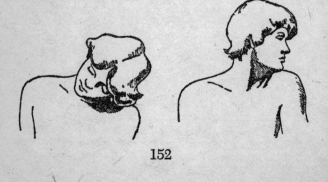

front of the body. Such deterioration can be large-ly prevented if one exercises these joints daily to keep the neck supple and mobile. You have only to have one episode of "wry neck" to realize how un-comfortable it is not to be able to bend the neck. Imagine sitting at a tennis match and having to turn your whole body to see the action or going duck hunting and having to lie on your back to get a shot at the ducks overhead.

The Squint

Squint your eyes tightly shut, then open them as wide as you can, even stretching the mouth open. (The jaw gets more than its share of exercise, especially in politicians, and needs no extra attention.)

Do the Squint whenever you feel like it, but only when you're alone. The Squint has subtle values. It exercises the muscles of the face, the mimetic muscles, making them more mobile and delaying the acquiring of wrinkles by keeping the muscles taut.

Exercise 19

The Lon Chaney

Make faces. That's right, all the faces you can. Contort your face, mouth and nose. Grimace. Look frightened. Look ugly. Make as many faces as you can, the most grotesque, misshapen faces you've ever seen.

This, like the Squint, also keeps the facial muscles tight and keeps them from sagging. It will keep you looking younger longer. Simple, isn't it?

Do these whenever you feel like it, and alone. Stop when your dog slinks away.

Deep Chest

(These exercises are more a collective routine than an actual "set" of exercises, owing to their simplicity and ease of performance. However, they are no less important than the "straining" we've been doing so far.)

Can breathing increase ROM and strengthen the muscles? No, not by itself. But Deep Chest, as I've described it here, definitely can. The tremendous forces that can be generated between the belly muscles and the diaphragm set up tensions in the back, thighs, across the chest and even in the shoulders. The muscles between the ribs are very strongly exercised this way. In fact, such breathing exercises can generate muscles as powerful as can be gotten in any other fashion. These, indeed, are super-exercises.

However, the Deep Chest routine is not to be associated with prolonged breath holding or with muscle strength. For this, we ask you to wait until you reach the S&S section. Breath holding, as we've pointed out in Chapter Six, is an extremely powerful way to bring forces to bear on your body that could be dangerous. So run through the Deep Chest routine once a day for at least two weeks before you advance to the S&S section.

These exercises will exercise the chest but will *not* increase the amount of air the chest will hold. They *will* increase the amount of air you can breathe in a minute, but only by a small percentage.

Exercise 20, therefore, is simply a deep breathing procedure, where you will fill your lungs completely, breathing in as deeply as you can, and then exhaling. When you think you've inhaled all you can, there is still more room—take in some more air! Then, exhale slowly, and force all the air possible out of your lungs.

All breathing exercises take breath away from the body and leave one light-headed. Do not hold these on the inhale for more than the count of two, at most. These are quite powerful and must be respected. Do all the Deep Chest exercises five times only.

Exercise 21. Breathe in again, deeply, and while the chest is full of air, raise the arms straight up and reach backwards as far as you can. This puts a real strain on the shoulders as the full chest opposes the motion of the arms. Even though the effort is very short, the chest and belly exercises are very powerful and can make the chest and belly very strong, very quickly.

Exercise 22. Now expel all the air from your chest, as you return to an upright position. Empty the lungs completely, sucking your belly in as far as it will go and forcing the last cubic centimeter of air out of your lungs.

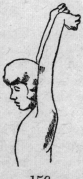

Exercise 23. Breathe normally for a few minutes. Then take another deep breath, as much as you can suck in, and force your belly outward as far as it will go, but resisting with your belly muscles as you do so, so that you aren't really distending your stomach. You will feel a great strain as you exert the belly muscles. Matching these two muscle systems against each other is matching two very strong and almost evenly matched antagonists. Not only can you learn better breathing, but you'll learn to hold your belly muscles in almost unconsciously.

Exercise 24. Inhale through your mouth, slowly, counting up to six as you do so. Now exhale just as slowly, but through the nose. Feel every motion of your chest as it moves from completely full to completely empty. Exhaling through the nose slows the motion of breathing, for the purpose of this exercise, and forces you to think about what is happening in your chest. Learning how it feels to breathe and learning to do it slowly is very good for control of muscles and, further, excellent for learning to relax. Anywhere you are, you can practice this slow breathing, with its attendant calming of the emotions.

The Bellywhoppers

Push your belly out against your belt as far as you can. Really stretch it. Now pull it in, until it seems to be flattened against your spine. Further. Actually try to suck your stomach in until you feel you could touch your spinal column with it. When it's in as far as it can go, take a deep breath, extending your belly outward again against your belt. Inhale as far as you can.

The intercostal and diaphragm muscles are driving the chest and, at this point, are maximally contracted. With the belly pushed outward, the belly wall muscles are relaxed. This is the easiest position in which to fill the chest.

Now continue as before, sucking in your belly, exhaling completely, getting all the air you can out of your lungs. Do this five times and rest.

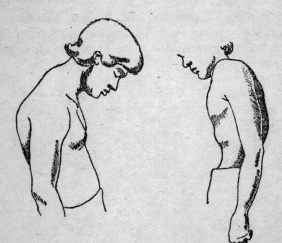

This pushing out and pulling in of the belly is one of the most beneficial exercises there are for flattening the gut. Not only is a big belly ugly to look at, it is also very unhealthy. It is uncomfortable and throws your posture off, thereby affecting the entire skeletal system. The minute you see someone with his belt hanging below his belly, you are looking at a man who will eventually have back problems. The only way he can carry that mass around in front of him and retain his balance is to bend his lower back and sling his shoulders backward. He is always tugging at that load. And as his belt flops lower and lower, he looks worse and worse.

These Bellywhoppers will keep your belly flat and trim.

Do as many as you want, until you feel the muscles starting to get sore. Each day try to do one more. You can do them sitting or standing, walking down the street, standing in elevators. They're not very visible at all. You might do them in the shower, reminding yourself each day as you lather your stomach. Then do as many as you want at any other time, also.

Spinal Lift #1

Lying on your back on the floor, lift your legs straight up without bending your knees. This is good for the stomach muscles, and it sounds like a strength and stamina exercise, but it is not. If you now put your hand under the lower part of your back, you will find it slips under easily; that is, the lower part of your back tends to lift off the floor in this position.

Now, lift your legs again, but make a conscious effort to keep the lower part of your back *on the floor.* Do the leg raises slowly, concentrating on keeping that portion of your back on the floor, lowering your legs and doing the exercise a few more times.

Remember this portion of your back during these and all types of "leg raise" exercises.

The iliopsoas muscle is the chief force in raising the legs. As it contracts, it pulls the lower spine forward and lifts it from the floor. Your hand will

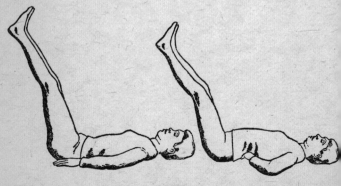

tell you this when you start to lift the leg. If you contract your muscles and keep your lower spine straight and *on* the floor, the legs will then be lifted partly by the belly muscles and only partly by the iliopsoas. This strengthens the belly muscles *and* the lower spine muscles that we are going to call on continually to strengthen your back and hold in your abdomen.

Do this and the next exercise five times, whenever you have time to stretch out on the living room floor.

Spinal Lift #2

If you found the previous exercise too difficult, i.e., if you couldn't get the lower back to stay on the floor, here's a way to accomplish it and derive a few extra benefits also.

Lie on the floor, as before, but this time draw up your knees, keeping your feet on the floor. Now lift your buttocks completely off the floor, so that you are supported only by your feet and shoulders. With one hand feel the spinal column where your upper back hits the floor, and *from the top down,* lower yourself to the floor *one vertebra at a time.* Feel each one make contact with the floor as you go, until you are again flat, with your entire spine on the floor.

Now do the leg raise again and see whether your lower back stays put. If not, keep trying it. This is an excellent exercise for women who desire not

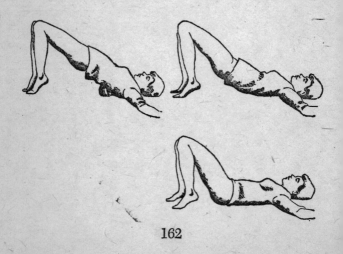

only better posture, but whose tummies need flattening. However, that can wait for the strength and stamina exercises. Right now we're interested in the ROM of your lower spinal column, and its proper position when you are erect. This exercise will improve the posture.

Back-to-the-Wall

I was once told by a balerina that ones balance was all in the small of the back. That seemed rather droll at the time, but I have since found that that is precisely where your center of balance is. Proper position of the low back is the most important single factor in our carriage, body balance and our whole attitude toward our own stance. Body balance, of course, is important in almost any sport.

These simple exercises for your pelvic ROM and proper carriage will make you walk, stand and look better all your life. First, they will get that forward bend out of the low back, and straighten it out. Second, they will get your pelvis tilted upward and that, in turn, will throw your weight more onto the balls of your feet, where it belongs. Third, they will strengthen your low back and belly muscles to help you maintain proper low back and pelvic positions. If you carry the positions you gain through these exercises into your daily life and activities, you will be amazed at how much easier they will be, how much less back pain you will have and how much better you will look. Oh yes—a good, fluid, *full* pelvic thrust will do wonders for your sex life.

Stand with your back to the wall, touching it with your heels and your head. Put your hand behind your back right at your belt line. Note how far your back is from the wall. It should be touching it.

Now try to tilt your pelvis enough to make your low back touch the wall, keeping your heels remaining against the wall. Try harder, perhaps bending the knees a bit. Work at this exercise whenever you feel like it, to get that pelvis tilted properly so that your low back touches the wall. This is the proper position of the pelvis. When you can do it, walk away from the wall keeping your pelvis in the same position. Notice that you now walk with your knees slightly bent, your belly pulled in and your pelvis tilted, your shoulders slightly forward in a balanced position. Even your fanny will have a tempting new curve to it, man or woman.

Your low spine is straight! You have achieved a relaxed position with all your muscles in proper position. Practice this every day and work very diligently to carry it through to every single one

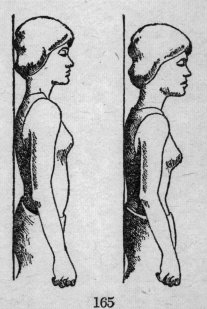

of your activities. Make everything you do a memory booster for Back-to-the-Wall. Eventually you will carry yourself that way without thinking about it, and you will have gained a great deal toward a firm and elastic body.

The Marrakesh Hot Dog

Lie on the floor, face up. Grasp your knees, the right knee with the right hand, left knee with the left hand. Now try to pull your knees straight into your armpits. At first, try to pull smoothly and evenly, but when your belly muscles stop hurting begin to pull harder. Even jerk the knees, if need be.

You will feel a strong pull across your back, strengthening the muscles around the sacrum. This is an excellent exercise for that low back pain that nags at you from time to time. I see a lot of this in the office, a very acute pain with a tender point located to either side of the sacrum. Cortisone injections usually help, but after having had it very badly myself and not willing to settle for shots the rest of my life, I got down on the floor and started jerking my knees hard into my armpits. In two minutes the pain had stopped, and the next time it returned I did the exercise again. Almost immediate relief. Now I do the exercise as a matter of routine, and have never had a recurrence of the low back pain.

Don't diagnose yourself, however. If your doctor

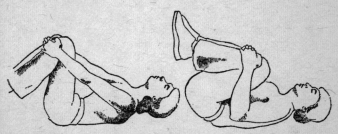

notices the tender points around your sacrum and is convinced it's nothing more serious than ligament strain or pulled muscles, try this exercise for it. Unfortunately, I have very little success getting patients to do it. They simply don't want to subject that already sore back to what appears to be an even more painful exercise. So they settle for the shots.

But for those of you with no back pain, do these as preventive medicine.

The Bobber

Simple. Sit on the edge of a chair with your legs apart and then bend over as far as you can with your arms crossed, try to touch your elbows to the floor. Relax slightly then really strain to get those elbows down. Bob up a little, get some momentum and bob down toward the floor. You will not be able to touch your arms to the floor, but in the course of trying you will pull your lower back as straight as it can get. Do five bobs per day and increase to ten.

This is actually an alternate to the Marrakesh Hot Dog and will strengthen the belly muscles, back muscles and shoulder muscles. Like the Marrakesh Hot Dog, it pulls the lower spine—in fact, the *entire* spine—into a smooth, C-shaped curve, where the nerve roots, which emerge from the back of the spine, are given maximum room and freedom for their motions. This is the best possible position to protect these delicate structures and to prevent pressure on them. Pressure on nerves, the so-called "disc syndrome," is one of the most excruciating pains perpetrated on the back. Every-

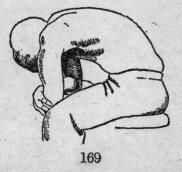

thing in the Retriever, the Marrakesh Hot Dog and Back-to-the-Wall is designed to encourage the spine into the C-shaped curve and thus prevent nerve compression and the acute agonies thereof.

The Ski Squat

At the Army and Air Force firing ranges, they call this the Philippine Squat, one of the basic rifle firing positions.

Squat on the floor with your heels *on the floor.* This is harder than it looks, and is a very good conditioning exercise for skiers. When you get down without your heels rising from the floor, keep going. Get down as low as you can, almost in a ball, all the while keeping your heels on the floor. You will eventually find, just as the people in primitive societies do, that it is a *very* comfortable position. Of course, our refined muscles and arteries will not tolerate this position for protracted periods, because our blood supply shuts off and our legs and feet grow numb. But young people and primitive people can sit this way for hours and find real comfort in it. Started at a young enough age, it could be carried into later life without distress, keeping the spine straight and tending toward that C-shaped curve.

Not only do primitive societies find the Ski

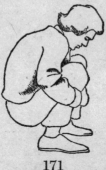

Squat position of maximum resting comfort, but they also find it one that is extremely practical to use. If the ground is cold or wet, the Ski Squat is an ideal way to relax. Also, childbirth is much easier in the Ski Squat position than in any other. Primitive peoples routinely give birth in this fashion and their incidence of birth complications is less than that of civilized peoples.

Obviously, this is not an exercise you can do just anywhere, but anytime your back bothers you, lock your office door, sneak off to the bathroom or find a quiet place in the house and sit this way for a while. It might, through regular use, save you a ruptured disc.

The Toe Touch

If there is anyone among us who hasn't heard of "touching the toes," he has been imprisoned in a closet for most of his life. However, this basic calisthenic is so standard, so simple and so *misunderstood,* that very few persons derive the proper benefit of it.

Mainly, people try to touch their toes to see whether they are "limber." Touch your toes, Joe. Can't? Sorry, you're in lousy shape. Can? Gee, you're in good shape, Joe.

But I'm saying it ain't so, Joe. Touching your toes does absolutely nothing for you unless you bend *backward* as far as you can *before* you touch your toes.

Stand erect. Throwing your hands up in the air, and then backward as far as they'll go, bend your torso backward and try to hang there for a few seconds. Bounce, if you can, gently, and then fling yourself forward and try to touch the toes. If you can't at first, don't worry. Even when you can't, you're deriving the same benefit as when you can. It's just that your spine isn't limber enough yet, that's all. But for every toe-touch you do, you must first bend *backward.* This is so that you can exercise those spongy pads between your vertebrae and keep the joints healthy and flexible. It stands to reason that if you only bend forward, eventually that's the *only* way you'll be able to bend.

Most yogis are fond of saying, "You're as young as your spine," and that seems to be a good rule of

173

thumb. Do five of the *proper* toe touches a day, and your spine will be young forever.

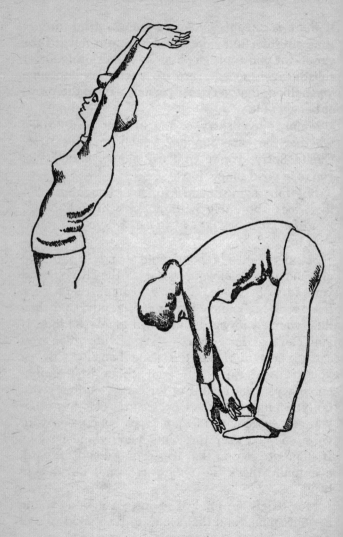

The Sidewinder

Stand erect, hands on your waist. Bend to the left side, stretching down as far as you can toward the ground. Then come up, slowly, and continue over to the right, repeating the stretch. Try to touch your elbows to the ground, which is impossible, but that's the direction to stretch in. Do as many of these as you can, and do them whenever you think of it. Remind yourself to do them every day, for they are extremely effective waist trimmers and are excellent for ROM of your spine.

A variation of this is to stand, hands on hips, and bend backward as far as you can, and rotate your upper body, making a circle using your waist as a fulcrum. Feel the waist muscles pulling as you rotate to the sides, your back as you rotate forward with the head down as far as possible, and your belly muscles as you return to the backward bend. All these muscles are tightening, pulling, to keep

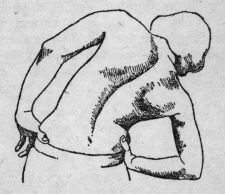

your sides, belly and other, inner muscles taut and trim.

In the process of this exercise, you are maintaining the full lateral or sideways motion of your spine. And you're strengthening the long muscles that lie on either side of the spine and the flank muscles that support the sides of your abdomen. This will effectively pull in your waist and trim off a half inch or so. Successive use of this, the Spinal Lift, the Marrakesh Hot Dog and the Retriever, will do wonders for your waist.

Perhaps the most common cause of sprains and ligament injuries across the back is weak back muscles and inadequate range of spine motion. Any activity requiring spinal strength *must* cause the spine bones to be compressed one upon the other. A supple spine with strong muscles holding it snugly together is the best protection. Think of your spine as an egg—it is common knowledge that a well-calcified chicken's egg cannot be broken by squeezing it end to end in the hand. Why is this? Because the pressure force across the egg is distributed smoothly along the shell and bent back on itself. The same thing pertains to your spine: when it is drawn tautly together and held by powerful muscles, it acts all of a piece, and is far more resistant to compressive and disruptive forces.

Ostrich Walk

While standing erect, strut in place, with each step raising the thigh as high as you can to touch your belly. You will quickly find this quite tiring, but it is very strengthening for such esoteric muscles as the psoas, iliacus, sartorius, rectus femoris and the great quadriceps. This ROM is essentially for the hip joints, stretching the hip capsule in the forward bending motion.

Do this for a dozen steps or so, increasing the frequency each day, being sure to pull the thigh against the belly with each step.

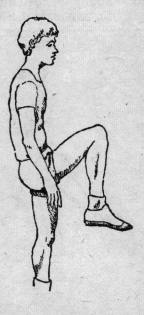

Point After Touchdown

Stand straight and stretch your leg backward as far as it will go, keeping the knee straight, as if you were getting ready to kick a football as far as you could. Stretch the leg so as to make the motion come from the hip joint instead of merely swinging your foot. Don't bend your back. When your leg is back as far as it can go, body straight, buttocks tight, suddenly swing your foot forward, kicking an imaginary football through the uprights. Swing your leg back down and do it again with the other leg. Do five of these, and add more daily.

This will accomplish essentially the same thing as the Ostrich Walk, i.e., loosen the hip joint to preserve the smooth, swiveling motion required of

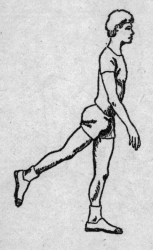

that ball-in-socket joint. The two exercises should be done together, one after the other, since they require a very short time span to perform, and can be done virtually anywhere.

Side, Kelly, Side!

Lie on your side. With your head resting on your extended arm, lift the leg straight up as far as it will go, keeping the knee straight. Try each time to raise it higher, lowering it slowly afterward. Reverse sides. This exercise is stretching the lateral muscles of the thigh, pulling them well out and rendering them flexible and supple.

It also exercises the tissue overlying the prominence we call the "hip," actually the greater trochanter of the femur. Each time you lift the leg you slide the skin and underlying tissues over this prominence. This helps prevent another kind of bursitis. The bursa between the greater trochanter and the skin is quite prone to irritation. This exercise will help prevent and even help cure this condition once it comes on. It also puts a good pull on the inside muscles of the thigh, the hamstrings that go from the pelvis to the femur. Keeping these

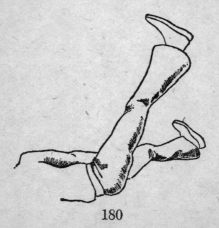

well stretched is excellent in preventing the contractures that prevent older people from separating their legs. Not designed as a power exercise, this one still gives good strength results, since lifting the mass of the leg by itself is hard work.

This has to be done in solitude and would be a good one to get out of bed with in the morning. Do as many as you can.

The Flamingo

While standing, bend your leg backward as far as it will go, flexing the knee. Finally, you will have to grasp your ankle and jerk the leg up further toward your thigh to get the last bit of motion out of it.

Return your foot to the floor and perform the maneuver with the other leg. Do this five times a day.

The last five or so degrees of motion of the knee joint is rarely achieved. It does not seem to matter a lot in ordinary life but this can be quite necessary after a knee injury and it certainly can do no harm to put this joint through its paces. In the process you are pulling the hip backward, extending it. When the hip freezes it does so by bending up on the belly and losing its backward bend. One

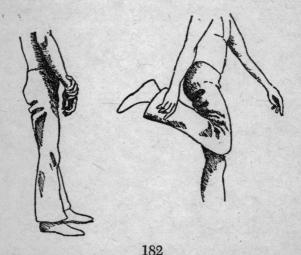

puts a strain on the hamstrings, the quadriceps and some on the gastrocnemius. If you can do this exercise without pulling on the leg with your hand, so much the better.

Anytime you're standing is a good time for the Flamingo. It looks like you are stretching.

The Ankle Roll

While sitting down, lift your foot clear of the floor and point your toes out as far as they'll go, straightening the ankle. Then bend the ankle back toward your head as far as it will go, and curl the toes simultaneously. Feel the muscles of the calf, the gastrocnemius and soleus pulling together.

Now gently roll your ankle through a full circle, in both directions. Do five of these a day, with both feet.

The gastrocnemius is obvious. It lies at the calf of the leg, in fact, it is called the "calf." It is the bulging mass that gets large and hard in runners and other types of athletes in whom running is important. Under it, or between it and the leg bones, is the soleus. This muscle has a large number of "white fibers" which means it can contract only slowly but it can hold a contraction longer and more easily than the gastrocnemius which has largely "red fibers." The ankle joint takes a merciless beating during the day. This quite small pivot of bone takes the entire weight of the body during

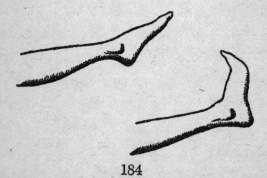

every activity from standing to violent changes of direction and torque during skiing and basketball. ROM done here daily will pay big dividends.

You can do these anytime you're sitting down. In fact, make sitting a memory crutch to doing these.

CHAPTER 9

The Strength and Stamina Exercises

Now we come to the part we've been working up to all along. This is the point at which we start to achieve additional strength and stamina. We call the biotonic maneuvers in this section "static thrust" exercises: "static" because you will be lifting no weights, in most cases moving no joints and in many cases not even moving the very muscles you are exercising; "thrust" because in each exercise the muscle has to be exerted, or "thrust" with all your power, against its tendons in order to gain additional strength. Remember that primarily you will be increasing your strength, and thereby gaining stamina, and you will begin feeling better *all the time.*

Your ROM exercises plus this added muscular conditioning will have a pronounced effect on your overall well-being, your vitality, your vim and

186

vigor—indeed, the very way you *feel* at the end of the day. You'll own more energy and alertness than you ever thought possible. Combined with the nutritional suggestions made earlier in this book, these exercises will make you physically sounder in almost every way—slimmer, trimmer, more attractive, stronger, more energetic and in possession of greater stamina that you've had at any time before in your adult life. *I promise!*

All the following exercises *can* be done repetitively and with less than maximum effort, but it will take longer for you to achieve your goal. I cannot stress too much the idea of performing each exercise to your *maximum*. Can't you hold a muscle as tense as you possibly can, for only six seconds?

By and large, we will be using one part of the body to oppose another; in other cases, a desk, a chair or a broom handle will act as the counterforce. At the start you may find a slow count of six is just too long, especially when you get a couple of days in and your muscles don't just whine but yell at you. Use a shorter count here, and settle for less than a maximum effort. Then, in the second and third week, really hit it!

Another point. It takes twenty times as long for a muscle to recover as it does for that muscle to contract. If you contract your biceps for six seconds it requires 120 seconds, or two minutes, for that muscle to recover, i.e., to build up its supply of ATP and refurbish its glycogen. Even a thirty-five percent contraction squeezes off the muscle's blood supply. Six seconds of contraction are six seconds with no oxygen to the muscle as the blood vessels collapse and no blood flows. So let your muscles relax between efforts and give them plenty of recovery time.

How do you know when you are really thrusting the muscle to its maximum capacity? When it hurts like hell, that's when. Your job is short, but it's painful. You have to make that muscle pull to the greatest extent you can for six seconds, which does hurt. But that's *all* you have to do.

Whereas I suggested the ROMs be performed several times, or as many as you wish, the strength and stamina exercises only have to be done *once a day!* And once you reach your goal, you only have to do them *once a week!* Imagine reaching the level of strength where you only have to do an exercise once a *week* to hold that muscle's maximum strength. Is it worth a try?

Okay, here we go . . .

The Claw

Holding your palm flat, and down, stretch the fingers out and apart as far as you can. Really stretch them. Hold the maximum stretch for a slow count of six. Then relax. Do it with your other hand.

This exercise stretches the extensor muscles of the hand and forearm, making your grip like that of a vise. People who show off by crushing unopened beer cans have achieved the strength of grip that this exercise will give you.

This is our first example of using one group of muscles to oppose another. The flexor and extensor muscles of the hand and forearm are opposing each other and being put under a great strain. Obviously the wrist and hand joint will be equally strained, tightened and drawn in.

Anytime you can do this is fine but you have to allow for the look of pain and tension on your face. You *cannot* do this exercise passively. You have to *look* like you're really working while you are at it.

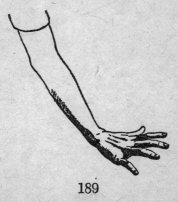

Fist of Mail

Make the tightest fist possible. Clench your fingers
into the tightest fist you've ever made, so much so
that your hand will start to tremble. If you have a
soft rubber ball, such as a handball, or tennis ball,
or small ball of yarn about two inches in diameter,
that will do fine to soften the exercise.

Concentrate on nothing but squeezing the ball
—real or imaginary—to smithereens. Concentrate
hard, gritting your teeth, grimacing. Count slowly
to six, and do it again with the other hand.

After twelve weeks, be very careful about shaking hands with people. The smart-ass who wants
to show off his "firm" handshake on you may end
up with broken fingers.

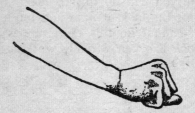

The Limp Wrist

Bend the wrist toward the forearm as hard as possible and to a slow count of six. This strengthens the flexor muscle of the forearm and the intrinsic muscles of the hand.

We have chosen to give you several different exercises to strengthen the wrist. You can do only one of these or you can do them all. Each one has a particular set of muscles that will be selectively strengthened, as with each one a particular set is put at such a position as to be maximally strained. Obviously, you will strengthen faster if you do all of these.

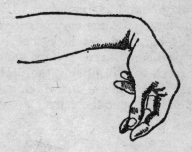

Exercise 42

The Power Fist

Clench the fist as hard as you can. Now, holding that clench with full power, bend the wrist backward. *It will hurt!* Adding the clenching of the wrist gives another dimension to the previous exercise, increasing power that doesn't occur in merely the wrist flexion. Be careful at the beginning of these two wrist exercises, as you will be putting great torque on the wrist joint.

These exercises, again, will improve your grip immensely, as well as adding strength and staying-power to your forearm, so important in many sports. There are many puny baseball players who have hit tremendously long home runs strictly because of wrist and forearm action. I have seen Hank Aaron hesitate to the very last second before swinging his bat, and yet flick that ball into a second tier pavillion. Boxers, golfers, tennis players, football players—they'll all sing the praises of the mighty wrist and forearm in bringing that extra measure of endurance to the game.

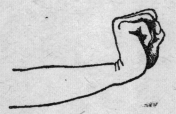

The Souper

With the elbow at right angles, turn the hand upward into supination, as though you were holding a small bowl of soup. Turn it up hard, and keep trying to turn it further outward for a slow count of six. You can use your other hand to oppose this motion, or you can grasp a broom handle braced between your knees.

This puts the supinator muscle, the forearm extensors and the biceps under a great strain, but its most important action is to get the last possible rotary motion from the head of the radius. As we pointed out before, this is the site of the infamous "tennis elbow."

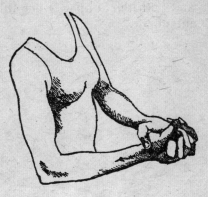

Thumbs Down

Keeping your elbow at right angles, turn your hand in the opposite direction used in the previous exercise, trying to achieve the classic "thumbs down" gesture. This time, however, if you are keeping your elbow strictly at a right angle, you'll find you can't go very far past the horizontal, much less achieve the vertical "down" position. Try hard, though, to get that thumb pointed directly at the floor. Both arms can be exercised at once, a saving of six whole seconds.

The best place for this exercise practice is, of course, at a sports event. Or when driving your car, sitting or reading, when the elbow is naturally bent.

This puts the pronator and extensor muscles under strain, and with the Souper is helpful in preventing "tennis elbow."

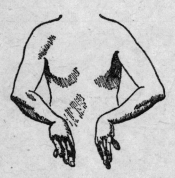

One-Man Indian Wrestle

Standing or sitting, bend the right elbow at a right angle. Clasp your left hand into your right hand, and bring the right hand up toward your right elbow, opposing the action with your left hand. The two will begin to struggle against each other. Increase the power of your right hand, trying to raise it to the shoulder, but not allowing it to move because of the opposing strength of the left hand. Hold for a slow count of six.

Office workers can do this at their desks *at least* once a day. As a variation, the office worker can slip one hand under his desk, and try to lift it; then try again with the other hand. The person at home can use his other hand, or an immovable object.

This exercise not only strengthens the biceps, but also brings the elbow into full flexion, something which seldom happens during the normal day for

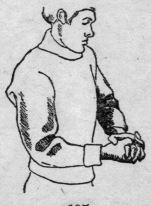

the average American. Even when we lift heavy things, we seldom lift *very* heavy things. As well as strengthening the biceps, the One-Man Indian Wrestle does wonders for the hand, forearm and shoulder muscles. Even the pectoral, trapezius and neck muscles are thrown into the fray.

The Poltergeist

This is an oldie but goodie. We did it as kids, and the odds are your own children have already discovered it. What has gone undiscovered is its beneficial results for shoulder and upper torso strength.

Stand with your side to a wall—close to it. Keeping your elbow straight, try to raise your arm by lifting out against the wall with the back of your hand, as if you were trying to lift your arm clear through the wall. Push very hard.

This puts a great force upon the deltoid and supraspinatus muscles. These are the only muscles in the shoulder that move the arm away from the body in a sideways motion. Every motion that lifts the arm away from the body uses these muscles, but we are seldom called upon to exert them against a great force.

As you suddenly step away from the wall and

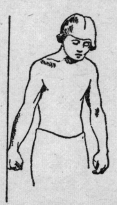

relax your arm, it will eerily rise against your will to almost level with your shoulders, as if a mischievous ghost were pulling at your arm.

The Bust-Buster

Extend your arms straight out, with palms together. Without bending your arms, squeeze your palms together, as if pushing one hand through the other. Squeeze hard. If you were to put a dynamometer between your hands you would see how little force you can muster in this position, but don't be discouraged by the lack of *apparent* force. You are working against a tremendous mechanical disadvantage. Almost three feet of arms are out there being pulled together only by the pectoralis major and minor muscles, which have only a very short hold on the bone. Feel for yourself—the muscles are attached only about two inches from the shoulder joint. That gives you a mechanical disadvantage of at least fifteen to one. However, your advantage physically is that the maximum effort here puts a far more powerful force *against* the muscle than it does in a situation when the advantage is *with* the muscle.

In other words, as you slowly bend your elbows and bring the hands closer to your chest, you will feel that you can exert more pressure as you

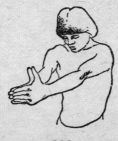

squeeze your palms together. This seems like you're doing much more good than before, but in fact you aren't. Have you ever noticed how much heavier things seem when held at arm's length? Case dismissed.

By the way, this exercise is the only one which conceivably could enlarge the apparent size of the female breast. I say "apparent" because the breast itself will not enlarge except under hormonal influences, but if the pectorals are enlarged it will certainly make the breast appear larger.

Self-Levitation

Sit on the floor between two straight chairs. Place your elbows one on each chair seat, legs straight in front of you. Now raise yourself up off the floor, lifting your buttocks. If this exercise seems too easy, place some heavy books or any other object on your lap. The idea here is to make it as difficult as possible, because a particularly powerful muscle is at work here, the latissimus dorsi. This muscle comes from the back and goes to the upper arm. It's the one the monkeys use to swing through the trees, and the one, when developed, that gives men that "triangular" look. Women needn't fear its overdevelopment.

This important muscle comes into play in such activities as climbing, tennis serves, throwing, swinging.

Do this exercise five times, and more as your strength develops. Because of the chairs and the

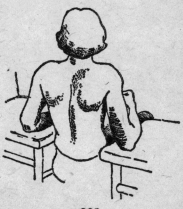

exertion required—especially if you use the books or other heavy object—you'll need some extra time to do it. Therefore, plan a specific time of the day, when you are usually alone and you can arrange for this exercise.

Ho-Hum

While standing or sitting, place the palm of the right hand behind your head, and try to pull it forward, while opposing the motion as hard as you can with the head. No motion should take place, but you will feel a tight strain on the neck muscles and the muscles of the upper arm, the triceps and biceps. The triceps, on the bottom of your arm as you extend it in front of you, is that muscle which grows flabby and saggy, especially in women, when you are out of shape.

This exercise is also very good for reducing tension headaches and pains in the back of the neck due to stress and strain at the office or when under other pressures.

Repeat the action with the left hand, and then perform it with both hands, reaching back in that "ho-hum" fashion as you would when sitting back to ponder a great thought or stretching back to relax after a long session of desk work.

Do each exercise to a count of six.

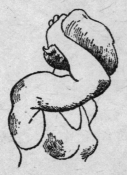

Oi Vey (or Mama Mia!)

This can be said to be the reverse version of the Ho-Hum. Place the palm of the hand against the forehead this time, and push back in the classic gesture of exasperation. Oppose the motion as hard as you can with the head. The same muscles as the Ho-Hum come into play, except with more emphasis on the muscles on the sides of the neck and the biceps.

Repeat with the other hand, and then do it briefly with both. If you are in public, pretend that you have been struck with a particularly deep thought, or else forgot something terribly important. You could also do a fine imitation of Rodin's *The Thinker*.

The Ho-Hum and the Oi Vey are good exercises for when you first sit down at a table or desk, such

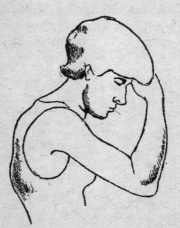

as that relaxing "all alone" cup of coffee in mid-morning, when you first get to work and start opening the mail, or anytime tension starts to develop in the back of the neck during tedious activities such as typing or writing.

The Sheboygan Shrug

This is another good exercise for dispelling tension or frustration, and will develop the trapezius very well. Sitting or standing, pull your shoulders upward in a great shrug, trying as hard as possible to tuck the head down and into your body as if you were a turtle. Really exert yourself—try to cover your ears with your shoulders, then drop them back to the normal position.

The trapezius muscle comes into play during this exercise as well as the muscles along the back of the neck. The beautiful contours on the top of the weight-lifter's shoulders are fleshed out trapezius muscles. Psychologically, this exercise is good for "shrugging off" worries and anxieties. It's no accident that every race I know of "shrugs off" its pressures.

You can do the Sheboygan Shrug almost any time of day, but late in the afternoon and early

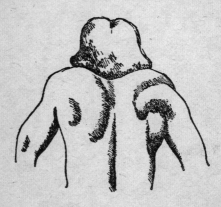

evening, when those daily tensions start to build up and the energy level starts to sag, is an excellent time. Also when reading, seated in waiting rooms, etc.

The Marilyn Monroe Come-Hither Shoulder Roll

This exercise is the classic satirical take off on "come hither" sexpots of cinema. Do the Sheboygan Shrug with only one shoulder, except this time rotate the shoulder in a complete circle, so that as you start with the shrug and roll the shoulder to the back, it lowers and will be fully dropped at the bottom of the rotation. Oppose the rotation strongly with the shoulder's own muscles as you do it. This flexes the shoulder and back muscles.

Repeat with the other shoulder, and then do it again with each shoulder.

This exercise is an excellent one for warming up before any sports activities in which bats or rackets are swung or balls are thrown.

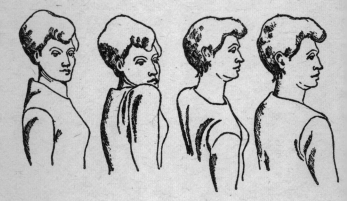

The Shoulder Squeeze

The shoulder squeeze is very good at board meetings when the board is getting bored. It is easy to do in public, too, because it looks exactly like you are just reminding yourself to stand or sit straight and are squaring your shoulders. Just pull your shoulders back and try to touch your shoulder blades together. As we did in the ROM exercise, imagine that you are trying to hold a coin between the blades.

This exercise stretches and flexes the rhomboid muscles, which are used in such activities as pulling the shoulders back and maintaining fine posture, as well as rowing, climbing, tennis and all sports in which the arm is pulled back often.

Do it several times a day, and you will find your posture improving daily.

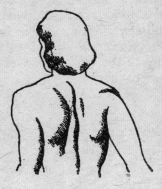

Pollywog Grunt

Lie on your stomach, clasping your hands together behind you on the small of your back. Now try to force your hands down toward your feet. As you struggle to force your hands down against those forces, a great many muscles are brought into play and exercised. These muscles are seldom exercised because of their location, but they are extremely valuable.

This exercise may not *feel* like you are accomplishing anything, but in fact you are putting a powerful strain on four of the greatest muscles of your back: the long muscles, the serratus anterior, the rhomboids and the latissimus dorsi. Also, all the shoulder muscles and even the muscles in the buttocks are exercised if this is done with maximum effort.

Be careful when you start this exercise, because it is *easy* to strain a muscle or two. However, after practice and a few weeks into the program, you definitely will start looking better from the rear.

This is a good exercise to remember when you are doing any of the other exercises that call for this position on the floor.

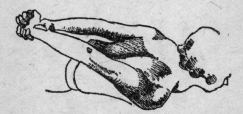

Parade Rest

While standing erect, put your hands behind your back in the classic "Parade Rest" position of your Army days. Ladies, ask your male friends the exact position—instead of the casual hands-behind-back position, the Parade Rest calls for the arms to be slightly lifted, so that your hands are tucked neatly into the small of your back, and the line from one forearm to the other is parallel to the ground.

Clasp your hands together and rotate them ninety degrees so that one palm is faced toward the floor, the other upward. Now try to push one palm down, while opposing it with an upward motion of the other. This is another exercise where you will feel that you have almost no power going for you, but again, this only means that the muscles involved are performing a great effort.

In Parade Rest, you are exercising the same muscles as in the One-Man Indian Wrestle, but now instead of the pectorals, you're bringing in the

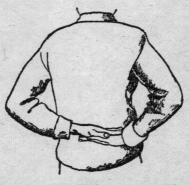

latissimus dorsi muscles most strongly. These muscles are useful in lifting, pushing, shoving, etc. and will improve your overall posture. Be sure to reverse your hands now and then.

Let it All Hang Out!

Here's another one of those embarrassing but important belly exercises.

Sitting down, have your belt snug but not tight. Ladies can put on a small belt from an outfit in the closet. Now push out your gut as far as it will go, pressing it strongly against the belt. Try to break the belt. Strain hard to enlarge the belly and hold it fully distended for a count of six and then relax.

I recommend doing this in the shower, whenever you begin washing your belly. Although you won't have a belt, you can perform this and the next exercise with no one watching. If you remind yourself every time you start lathering up the mid-section, fairly soon a Pavlovian reaction will set in and you'll be doing these every day, regardless of how busy you are. The dramatic results will be felt

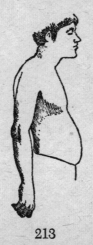

very soon, perhaps the first week of the program.

We may as well name the belly muscles for you now, since they will be serving you well in the coming weeks, holding your belly flat and transforming you into a svelte, athletic-looking person. They are the external and internal oblique, the rectus abdominis and the transversalis. Remember that any exercise of the belly strengthens the diaphragm, and therefore the chest.

You Leave Me Breathless!

When you have become fairly adept at Let It All Hang Out!, try this one and eventually do them together. This is essentially the same as LIAHO! except that before you push out your belly against the belt, expel all the air from your lungs. Hold the lungs empty for as long as you can and strain the gut outward against your belt. Hold it for the count.

This moves the same set of muscles as LIAHO! We include it because it does something LIAHO! does not: it forces the belly muscles to work at a severe mechanical disadvantage. Without the downward thrust of the diaphragm pushing on the bowels, the belly muscles have a difficult time forcing themselves outward.

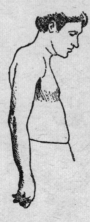

Look, Ma, No Hands!

This is a variation of the Flamingo in the ROM section, except that this time no helping out with your hands is allowed. Thigh muscles only are used.

Standing erect, lift one thigh up and inward toward the belly, trying to tuck it right up there against your gut. Remember, no hands. Use the thigh muscles alone, and pull hard. The iliopsoas, the sartorius and the great quadriceps are being strengthened. Because the quadriceps are the most powerful muscles in the body, there is no need to explain their importance in running, jumping, lifting, moving swiftly and easily to either side, hiking and practically everything you ever do with your thigh muscles.

Do the exercise again with the opposite leg. Try it sitting down, too, just for variety.

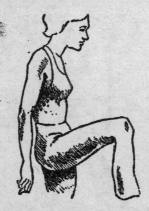

The Sidestepper

This is the leg version of the Poltergeist. Stand sideways to a wall, and with your foot push against the wall as if you were going to lift your leg out to the side. Strain hard against the wall, keeping the leg very straight and your knee locked. The power for this exercise will come directly from the hip, and you'll be working at a great mechanical disadvantage.

Hold the maximum strain against the wall for the count, and step away. You'll find that pesky little poltergeist trying to lift your leg against your will, just as with the arm exercise.

This will strengthen your tensor fascia latae, the vastus lateralis and gluteus minimus muscles, and give you additional strength for those activities requiring leg power and quick lateral movements.

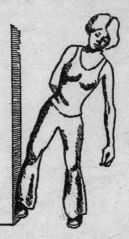

The Locust

The Locust is one of the classic yoga positions and probably the best exercise you'll ever do for your entire low back-spine-belly-thigh-fanny-system. Lie on the floor face down, belly flat against the floor. Place your hands under you, so that the palms cup your pubic bone or lower abdomen, out of the way. Keeping your knee locked and leg straight, lift your thigh as high off the floor as you can, being careful to keep the pubic bone on the floor (the hand contact will monitor this for you.) Lift it slowly, and hold it for the count, then lower it slowly. Alternate legs, and eventually do it with both legs at once.

This marvelous exercise stretches, flexes and strengthens the many extensor muscles of the hip, such as the gluteus maximus and the biceps femoris. It is also remarkably good for contracting the fanny and strengthening the low back area, keeping your spine supple and flexible.

Eventually you will find yourself performing this exercise easily and quite dramatically. When you feel this confidence, double your efforts to

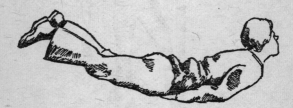

raise the leg as high as possible, even trying to double them back over your head, but without unlocking the knees. You'll be surprised at how proficient you will become.

Knee Squeeze

Lying on your back, bring the knee up as far as you can to your chest, without the aid of your hands (as in the ROM exercises). This can be said to be the prone version of the Look, Ma, No Hands! and will strengthen your leg muscles. Alternate legs, and finally try to pull the knees as far as you can toward your chest or, for that matter, toward your forehead if you'd like to raise your head, neck and upper back at the same time.

Do this alone for the first few days, as an added but potentially embarrassing benefit is the rapid and noisy relieving of trapped gas in your bowels.

The Knee Squeeze is also good for the strength in the lower back and stomach muscles.

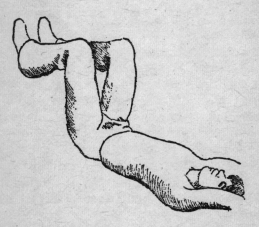

The Sit-Kicker

Here's another excellent one for the overweight people of the world, especially the obese. For some reason which the medical world isn't quite sure of yet, the knees seem to take all the abuse of being overweight. Because they are bearing all the weight and trying to maintain motion at the same time, the hip, ankle and foot joints are also stressed, but the knee takes all the knocking, developing arthritis and eventually disintegrating into nothing but a jointful of broken bones, causing almost total immobility.

Sit straight in a chair. Slowly lift your right leg, toes pointing out, which is to say straightening the knee joint. As you get higher, curl the toes down toward the floor. Strain hard. If you're doing it right you will feel the other leg contracting, too, and perhaps you may cramp at first in your calf muscles. After the count, curl your toes the opposite way. Strain hard to lift that leg high!

This strong knee exercise pays off in many ways. Besides preventing some of the arthritis that the knee will develop as you grow older (or has developed already because you are overweight), this exercise will strengthen almost every muscle of the leg, hip, ankle and foot, particularly the quadriceps, and will pull the knee joint tight. Nothing will ever serve a person better than the quadriceps muscle, and the static thrust of this simple knee extension will build that powerful muscle admirably.

When the leg muscles are strong, one has a springing, snappy gait with a good, strong stride.

These can help put the foot in proper place for walking. But if these are weak, the foot may drag and this could be one of the contributing factors to the breaking of the hip. Walking arcoss a rug or up a step may cause tripping as the foot gets in the way. The subsequent fall may then cause the hip to snap.

A further advantage to foot exercises is keeping the feet healthy so the owner can wear shoes of his or her choice. Ugly, malformed toes, weak arches and weak leg muscles can make it impossible to wear high arch shoes or shoes with narrow toes. Vanity itself is served in keeping the feet supple.

If the quadriceps and the hamstring muscles are kept powerful, the knee is protected and all usual activities are possible. Climbing stairs is an agony to one with weak quadriceps. We have all seen the

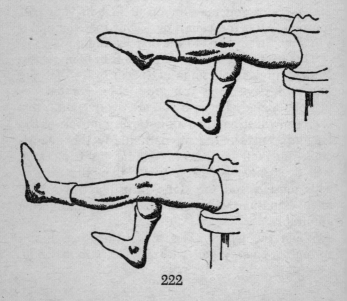

poor soul going up one stair at a time because his thighs were too weak for the smooth effort of climbing. Even more dramatic is the difference the patient in a cast shows. It is not at all unusual for a thigh to lose two inches in circumference when it is immobilized in a cast. The cast is removed and that flimsy muscle cannot do the work required to hold the knee and the patient has real trouble. But if he has done his exercises as directed here, he can come out of the cast with a thigh as strong as the opposite side and be quite ready for walking.

Another powerful reason for keeping the thighs strong is bending forward. If the thighs are weak one must bend with the back—an excellent way to strain it and end up in much pain. Strong thighs allow one to bend with the legs, the safe way to bend over.

The Wholistic Stretch

Here's where you take over an entire doorway for a few moments. Stand in the doorway, as you did on that bathroom scale to measure your strength, and push up hard with both hands against the top of the jamb. Use a stool or a few books if you can't reach the top of the doorway. Try to push it through the roof, with your feet standing on their toes to help you gather force to push that jamb.

Next put your hands on the sides of the doorway, and try, Samson-like, to demolish the entire doorway. Exert yourself hard to push the sides of the doorway completely apart. Hold each strain for the count and relax.

Do these every time you go through a doorway

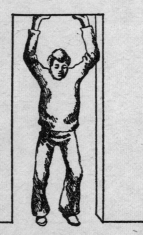

and you will notice striking results within the first week. Almost every large muscle of the body, and many, many small ones, will be called upon during these two exercises.

The Pelvic Pull-Up

Lie on your back, knees flexed. Put your hand under the small of the back, and then bend your back until the hand is being squeezed. You can accomplish this by rotating the pelvis forward. Feel the lower spine shift, until it finally traps your hand underneath. Squeeze the hand very hard, and hold it for the count. As you progress in this, you will learn to bend your back into the proper position without bending your knees, getting all the straightening of the back with the pelvic tilt alone.

This exercise is a variation of the Spinal Lifts #1 and #2, and the Back-to-the-Wall, but is far less strenuous in case you found the others a bit much at first. As with the others, it will greatly benefit your back, posture and your belly muscles.

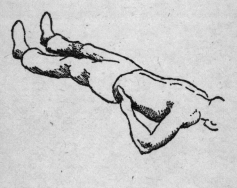

The Peruvian Shoulder Buster

Sit on the floor in front of a chair. Reach back with your hands and try to place your palms on the seat of the chair, so that you can raise yourself off the ground in kind of a reverse push-up. If you can, hold yourself in the full "up" position for the count, and then slowly lower yourself.

Many people, perhaps most, will have to begin this in the "up" position and lower themselves to the floor, keeping their hands on the seat of the chair. We strongly recommend this! Do not do this exercise starting from the "down" position until you have twenty-one consecutive performances from the "up" position under your belt, or unless you are in exceptionally fine shape to begin with. Reaching up behind for the chair seat puts a maximum disadvantage on the shoulder, and a severe

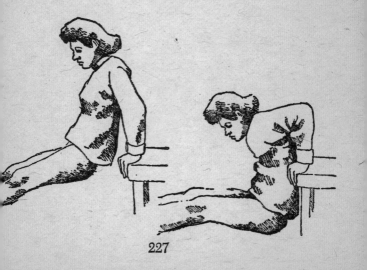

strain can result when an effort is made to raise the body.

This is a fine exercise for shoulders and back, as well as the arms and the backs of the legs. It's an excellent overall toner for most athletic activities, and if the exercise itself doesn't cause a muscle pull or a sprain, it will prevent these from happening in the future.

The Nadia Comanici Toner

Like the Wholistic Stretch, this is designed as the ultimate belly exercise which will also benefit the entire body, toning up all sorts of muscles and ligaments. Lie on the floor, face up. Now do a half sit-up, while at the same time raising your legs into a half leg-raise, forming a "V" with your body. Reach for but do not grab your knees. Hold this for the count. Eventually, you should be able to achieve a full ninety-degree shape as you learn to raise your head and legs higher.

Almost every muscle in your body is being used in this exercise, and in fact if you could accomplish it right off you were in pretty good shape to begin with. It is far more difficult than it sounds, as you'll soon find out. But it is one of the best exercises you can do, especially for the belly and leg muscles. You may not wind up with Nadia's talents, but you will have a fine firm belly.

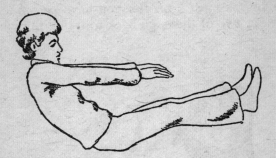

The Classic Push-Up

We end the program with the classic push-up. It is included primarily as a measure of your progress, and we suggest you do it but once a week to check on how far you have come. Doing all the other exercises should make you able to get down and perform a number of push-ups far greater than you could when you first started the program.

But do them properly. Lying face down, legs out straight, place your palms directly under your shoulders. Keeping your entire backbone straight, and without bending your head backward in the slightest, lift your entire stiff body off the floor. Do not bend your knees. When raised, the only parts of you that should be touching the floor are the toes and your hands.

Persons finding this too difficult at first may raise themselves for a week or two only from the knees. That is, keeping your knees on the floor, raise yourself up as before. This reduces the amount of weight you must lift. After you have performed a week or two of these, go back to trying the whole

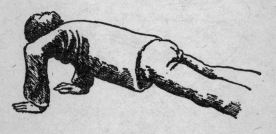

push-up. Your arms and chest may have developed enough to get you at least through one of them. But remember, no belly sagging, no neck bending. Keep the entire spine perfectly straight.

Figure 4

Popular Recreational Activities of America and the Exercises That Will Increase Proficiency and Stamina

tennis, handball, squash, racquetball	Claw; Fist of Mail; Limp Wrist; Power Fist; Souper; Thumbs Down; Bust-Buster; Self-Levitation; Pollywog Grunt; You Leave Me Breathless!; Sit-Kicker; Wholistic Stretch.
golf	Sit-Kicker; Thumbs Down; Souper; One-Man Indian Wrestle; Poltergeist; Marilyn Monroe Come-Hither Shoulder Roll; Shoulder Squeeze; Parade Rest; Let It All Hang Out!; Peruvian Shoulder Buster.
hiking	Sit-Kicker; Deep Chest; You Leave Me Breathless!; Look, Ma, No Hands!; Sidestepper; Locust; Wholistic Stretch.
sailing	Sit-Kicker; Claw; One-Man Indian Wrestle; Power Fist; Shoulder Squeeze; Pollywog Grunt; Let It All Hang Out!; Peruvian Shoulder Buster.
skiing	The skier should do as many of the S&S exercises as he can, and as often as he can. We especially recommend the Nadia Comanici Toner and the Sit-Kicker.
softball, football	Sit-Kicker; Claw; Souper; Thumbs Down; One-Man Indian Wrestle; Bust-Buster; Ho-Hum; Oi Vey; Pollywog Grunt; You Leave Me Breathless!; Wholistic Stretch; Sidestepper.
bowling	Sit-Kicker; Peruvian Shoulder Buster; Look, Ma, No Hands!; Locust; Nadia Comanici Toner; One-Man Indian Wrestle.
climbing	Sit-Kicker; Claw; Fist of Mail; Limp Wrist; Power Fist; Souper; Thumbs Down; Self-Levitation; Sheboygan Shrug; Pollywog Grunt; You Leave Me Breathless!; Look, Ma, No Hands!; Knee Squeeze.
soccer	Back Scratcher; Deep Chest; Let It All Hang Out!; Sidestepper; Sit-Kicker; Nadia Comanici Toner.
basketball	Clutch; Tennis Non-Elbow; Confidence Strut; Deep Chest; Fist of Mail; Bust-Buster; You Leave Me Breathless!; Sit-Kicker, Classic Push-Up.

swimming	Confidence Strut; Wrist Twist; Deep Chest; Spinal Lift #1; Marrakesh Hot Dog; One-Man Indian Wrestle; Poltergeist; Self-Levitation; Pollywog Grunt; Knee Squeeze.
jogging	Fist Wrist Twist; Let Your Fingers Do the Walking; Deep Chest; Wholistic Stretch.

---

*N.B.: Every sport requires all ROM exercises every day.

Bibliography

Altschule, M. D. *The Medical Clinics of North America.*
Volume 58, No. 2. Philadelphia: W. B. Saunders Co.,
1974.

Best, C. H., and Taylor, H. B. *The Physiological Basis
of Medical Practice.* Eighth Edition. Baltimore: The
Williams and Wilkins Co., 1966.

Currier, Dean P. Ph. D. "Maximal Isometric Tension of
the Elbow Extensors at Varied Positions. Part I. As-
sessment by Cable Tensiometer." *Physical Therapy.*
Volume 52(10):1043–1049. October 1972.

Hellebrandt, F. A. "Application of the Overload Prin-
ciple to Muscle Training in Man." *American Journal
of Physical Medicine.* Volume 37:278–283. 1958.

Huxley, H. E. "The Mechanism of Muscular Contraction." *Scientific American.* Volume 213(6):18–27. De-
cember 1965.

Key, J. A. and Conwell, H. E. *The Management of Fractures, Dislocations and Sprains.* Pages 1014–1020. St.
Louis: C. V. Mosby Co., 1956.

Krusen, Frank H., M.D., Kottke, Frederic J., M.D., and Ellwood, Paul M., Jr., M.D. *Handbook of Physical Medicine and Rehabilitation.* Philadelphia: W. B. Saunders Co., 1966.

Liberson, W. T. "Brief Isometric Exercises." Chapter Twelve in *Therapeutic Exercise,* edited by Sidney Licht, M.D. Second Edition. 1965. Published by Elizabeth Licht, 306 Fountain St., New Haven, Conn. Pages 307–326.

Lighthill, Sir James. "Atherogenesis Initiating Factors." Ciba Foundation Symposium 12. New York: Elsevier, 1973.

Magness, John I., M.D., Lillegard, Carol, R.P.T., Sorensen, Signia, R.P.T., and Winkowski, Peggy, R.P.T. "Isometric Strengthening of Hip Muscles Using a Belt." *Archives of Physical Medicine and Rehabilitation.* Volume 52(4):158–162. April 1971.

Moore, J.C., Ph.D. "Active Resistive Stretch and Isometric Exercise in Strengthening Wrist Flexion in Normal Adults." *Archives of Physical Medicine and Rehabilitation.* Volume 52(6):264–269. June 1971.

Mueller, Erich A., M.D. "Influence of Training and of Inactivity on Muscle Strength." *Archives of Physical Medicine and Rehabilitation.* Volume 51(8):449–461. August 1970.

Watson-Jones, Sir Reginald. *Fractures and Joint Injuries.* Volume 1, Fourth Edition. Pages 153–156. Baltimore: The Williams and Wilkins Co., 1955.

INDEX

THE BEST OF THE BESTSELLERS
FROM WARNER BOOKS!